THE MEANING
OF MADNESS

True, we love life, not because we are used to living, but because we are used to loving. There is always some madness in love, but there is also always some reason in madness.

—Friedrich Nietzsche, *Thus Spake Zarathustra*

THE MEANING OF MADNESS

NEEL BURTON

Acheron Press

Flectere si nequeo superos
Acheronta movebo

© Acheron Press 2015

Published by Acheron Press

All rights reserved. No part of this book may be reproduced or transmitted, in any form or by any means, without permission.

A CIP catalogue record for this book is available from the British Library.

ISBN 978 0 9929127 3 4

Typeset by Phoenix Photosetting, Chatham, Kent, United Kingdom
Printed and bound by SRP Limited, Exeter, Devon, United Kingdom

About Neel Burton

Dr Neel Burton is a psychiatrist, philosopher, writer, and wine-lover who lives and teaches in Oxford, England.

He is the recipient of the Society of Author's Richard Asher Prize, the British Medical Association's Young Authors' Award, the Medical Journalists' Association Open Book Award, and a 'Best in the World' Gourmand Award.

www.neelburton.com

About Acheron Press

Acheron Press was established in 2008 by Neel Burton for the purpose of producing and publishing challenging, thought-provoking books without the several constraints of a commercial, sales-driven approach.

The name 'Acheron' was inspired by a verse from Virgil's *Aeneid*:

Flectere si nequeo superos, Acheronta movebo

The line is often translated as, 'If I cannot bend Heaven, I shall move Hell', and was chosen by Freud as the epigraph to his *Interpretation of Dreams*.

According to the psychoanalyst Bruno Bettelheim, the line encapsulates Freud's theory that people who have no control over the outside world turn inward to the underworld of their own minds.

Contents

Preface to the Second Edition

This second edition aims to return *The Meaning of Madness* to relevancy by reflecting recent changes in the landscape of psychiatry and mental health, including the latest research and statistics and the advent of DSM-5.

I have also taken the opportunity to rework the text, and, while the structure has not sensibly changed, I hope that the arguments are more forceful and finely articulated than in the first edition.

Finally, responding to requests from students and course leaders, I have added a comprehensive index and full set of references.

Neel Burton
Oxford, October 2015

Introduction

In the UK, mental ill health is recognized as the single largest cause of disability, contributing almost 23 per cent of the disease burden and costing over £100 billion ($157 billion) a year in services, lost productivity, and reduced quality of life. Every year in the EU, about 27 per cent of adults are affected by mental disorder of some kind. In the US, almost one in two people will meet the criteria for a mental disorder in the course of their lifetime. Data from the US National Health Interview Survey indicate that, in 2012, 13.5% of boys aged 3-17 had been diagnosed with attention deficit hyperactivity disorder (ADHD), up from just 8.3% in 1997.

There is no denying that a lot of people are suffering. But are they really all suffering from a mental disorder, that is, a medical illness, a biological disorder of the brain? And if not, are doctors, diagnoses, and drugs necessarily the best response to their problems?

Since 1952, the number of diagnosable mental disorders has burgeoned from 106 to over 300, and now includes such constructs as 'gambling disorder', 'minor neurocognitive disorder', 'disruptive mood dysregulation disorder', 'premenstrual dysphoric disorder', and 'binge-eating disorder'.

According to a recent report, antidepressant prescriptions in England rose from 15 million items in 1998 to 40 million in 2012, this despite the mounting evidence for their ineffectuality. Selective serotonin reuptake inhibitors (SSRIs) in particular have become something of a panacea, used not only to treat depression, but also to treat anxiety disorders, obsessive-compulsive disorder, and bulimia nervosa, and even some physical disorders such as premature ejaculation in young men and hot flushes in menopausal women. In the UK, the SSRI fluoxetine is so commonly prescribed that trace quantities have been detected in the water supply.

But despite all this apparent progress in diagnosis and treatment, people who meet the diagnostic criteria for such a paradigmatic mental disorder as schizophrenia tend to fare better in resource-poor countries, where human distress can take on very different forms and interpretations to those outlined in our scientific classifications.

Psychiatry is in a crisis precipitated by its own success, and, assuming that it once did, the medical or biological model is no longer helping. The specialty of the heart is cardiology, the specialty of the digestive tract is gastroenterology, and the specialty of the brain is neurology and psychiatry. But neurology is not psychiatry, which literally means 'healing of the soul'.

Some mental disorders undeniably have a strong biological basis, but even these have many more aspects and dimensions than 'mere' physical disorders.

This book aims to open up the debate on mental disorders, to get people interested and talking, and to get them thinking. For example, what is schizophrenia? Why is it so common? Why does it affect human beings but not other animals? What might this tell us about our mind and body, language and creativity, music and religion? What are the boundaries between mental disorder and 'normality'? Is there a relationship between mental disorder and genius? These are some of the difficult but important questions that this book confronts, with the overarching aim of exploring what mental disorders can teach us about human nature and the human condition.

The first five chapters treat of common mental disorders, and the sixth is on the topic of suicide and self-harm. Ideally, the chapters ought to be read from first to last, but they can also be read as stand-alone essays. Each of the chapters assumes little prior knowledge of the mental disorder under consideration, and begins by furnishing a brief, textbook-like description of the forms that it takes. This enables the reader not only to learn about the mental disorder, but also to engage with the broad discussion that follows. The first chapter, 'Personality and personality disorders', is exceptional in that it begins with a discussion of what makes a person a person, and of the extent to which a person can be held responsible for who he is.

I hope you enjoy the read.

'In that direction,' the Cat said, waving its right paw round, 'lives a Hatter: and in that direction,' waving the other paw, 'lives a March Hare. Visit either you like: they're both mad.'
'But I don't want to go among mad people,' Alice remarked.
'Oh you can't help that,' said the Cat: 'we're all mad here. I'm mad. You're mad.'
'How do you know I'm mad?' said Alice. 'You must be,' said the Cat, 'or you wouldn't have come here.'

—Lewis Carroll, *Alice's Adventures in Wonderland*

Chapter 1

Personality and
personality disorders

For dust thou art,
and unto dust shalt thou return.

—Genesis 3:19 (KJV)

On September 13, 1848, one Phineas Gage was working on the construction of the Rutland and Burlington Railroad when he accidentally ignited some gunpowder with a large tamping iron. The iron was blown through his head (Figure 1.1) with such force that it landed several yards behind him.

Although Gage survived and was even talking and walking moments after the accident, his friends described him as 'no longer Gage'. The local doctor, JM Harlow, later reported in the *Boston Medical and Surgical Journal* that:

> Gage was fitful, irreverent, indulging at times in the grossest profanity (which was not previously his custom), manifesting but little deference for his fellows, impatient of restraint or advice when it conflicts with his desires, at times pertinaciously obstinate, yet

capricious and vacillating, devising many plans of future
operations, which are no sooner arranged than they are abandoned
in turn for others appearing more feasible. A child in his
intellectual capacity and manifestations, he has the animal passions
of a strong man. Previous to his injury, although untrained in the
schools, he possessed a well-balanced mind, and was looked upon by
those who knew him as a shrewd, smart businessman, very
energetic and persistent in executing all his plans of operation. In
this regard his mind was radically changed, so decidedly that his
friends and acquaintances said he was 'no longer Gage'.

The case of Phineas Gage raises a number of important questions about personality. What is the nature of personality? What is it that makes you who you are, and what would it take to make you someone different? What is a personality disorder, and, conversely, is there such a thing as an ideal personality? Is an ideal personality possible or even desirable?

In *The Development of Personality*, psychiatrist Carl Jung (1875-1961) emphatically described personality as 'the supreme realization of the innate idiosyncrasy of a living being... an act of high courage flung in the face of life, the absolute affirmation of all that constitutes the individual, the most successful adaptation to the universal conditions of existence coupled with the greatest possible freedom for self-determination'. More prosaically, personality can simply and effectively be defined as a person's pattern of thinking, feeling, and behaving. This pattern is formed from an early age, and, once formed, is both pervasive and enduring.

The term 'personality' derives from the Ancient Greek *persona*, meaning 'mask'. In all human civilizations, masks are used both to

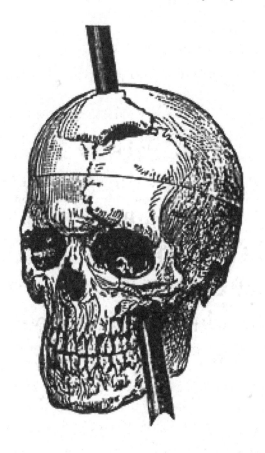

Figure 1.1. The iron bar passed through the ventromedial areas of the prefrontal cortex of the brain. From Harlow JM (1868): *Recovery from the passage of an iron bar through the head*. Publications of the Massachusetts Medical Society 2:327-347.

disguise and to reveal—albeit in a restricted or caricatured manner— the personality of their bearers. This dual function of masks is brought out in a painting by James Ensor (1860-1949), *Self-Portrait with Masks* (see book cover). This striking piece of art seems to invite us to reflect on the nature of our personality, and perhaps also to compare it to that of the Artist, who is stereotypically unburdened by social and cultural expectations and the falsehood and hypocrisy that they often entail. The Artist alone has the courage to be.

According to philosopher Søren Kierkegaard (1813-1855), to be a 'particular individual' is 'the only true and highest significance of a human being, so much higher as to make every other significance illusory'. Whatever one may feel about this pronouncement, it is difficult to imagine meeting someone who did not have any personality at all. Such an individual would, if anything, be little more than a random collection of thoughts, feelings, and behaviours, and without any meaning, purpose, or direction. This suggests that personality is not merely an optional adornment or embellishment that we carry around to make ourselves seem more interesting or appealing. Rather, personality is at the very core of our concept of personhood, perhaps even approximating or equating to personhood.

While it is difficult to imagine what it might be like for someone not to have any personality at all, it is, perhaps, just about possible to imagine what it might be like if everyone had the same—exactly the same—personality. In this scenario, our interactions with others would lose much of their purpose and attraction, and any meaningful and fulfilling relationship would be at best difficult and at worst impossible. If we feel that such a life would be less worthwhile, then this might tell us something about what does make life worthwhile. Philosopher Jean-Paul Sartre (1905-1980) famously held that 'hell is other people', but perhaps so too is heaven, and herein lies all the problem.

Non-human entities such as my neighbour's cat, the rosebush in the garden, or the weather do not have a personality (or at least a human personality) like you or me. Yet we have a strong tendency to anthropomorphize them, that is, to lend them a human personality, because this helps us to interpret them and relate to them. Following through with this thought, anthropomorphizing the universe produces our concept of God, a generally benevolent man with a white beard and sandals, not too dissimilar from Plato or Aristotle, whom we find easier to understand and relate to than dark and infinite cosmos—and who, we say, created us in his own image!

In light of this discussion, it appears that Kierkegaard's pronouncement that to be a 'particular individual' is 'the only true and highest significance of a human being' is both correct and self-evident— self-evident because a human being can only be a particular individual if he is to be anything meaningful at all. Taking this line of reasoning one step further, the more we develop and express our unique selves, the more organized and meaningful we become.

Personality is defined as a person's pattern of thinking, feeling, and behaving. All well and good, but what happens if we dig deeper? What is a 'person', and, more pointedly, what does it take for a person no longer to be that same person? Are you the same, identical person at all times? Are you the same person that you were a minute, a day, a year, or ten years ago? If so, what do you have in common with the person that you were then?

A person is a mental being, but not just any mental being, because many animals are also mental beings. A person is a self-conscious mental being who, according to philosopher John Locke (1632-1704), is 'a thinking, intelligent being, that has reason and reflection, and can consider itself as itself, the same thinking thing, in different times and places'. Thus, you are a person because you can think about yourself in the past, future, and conditional, and in a variety of different settings: 'Next February I might go on a holiday to India', 'Last summer I went on holiday to Spain', 'Last week I could have won the lottery, if only I had bought a ticket'.

If a person is a 'self-conscious mental being', what is it that makes him so? Is it his body, his brain, his soul? Imagine that he has a serious accident that leaves him lying brain-dead on a hospital bed. His body is still alive, but he is no longer self-conscious nor can he ever again be. Is he then still a person? If not, his physical body is not what makes him a person.

Let us for a moment turn to the second aspect of the question, *what does it take for a person no longer to be that same person?* Some have argued that a person at a time A can be the same as a person at a time B because his body or brain is the same body or brain at both times, in the sense that they are spatiotemporally continuous, that is, continuous in time and space. Others have argued that they are the same not because they are spatiotemporally continuous, but because they are psychologically continuous in that the mental state of the person at a time B derives or descends from the mental state of the person at a time A.

To help elucidate this problem, philosopher Sydney Shoemaker (born 1931) asks us to imagine that science has progressed to such an extent that brain transplants have become possible. Two men, Mr Brown and Mr Robinson, each have their brains removed and operated on at the same time. However, a poorly trained assistant inadvertently places Brown's brain into Robinson's skull, and Robinson's brain into Brown's skull. One of these two men dies, but the other—let's say the one with Brown's brain and Robinson's body—eventually regains consciousness. When asked his name, this entity—let us call him 'Brownson'—replies, 'Brown'. When Brown's wife and children walk in, he recognizes them, and is able to recollect events from Brown's past.

Who then is this man Brownson with Brown's brain and Robinson's body? If he is Brown, as most people would argue, then a person cannot be reduced to a body, as the above brain-dead scenario may already have suggested. This leaves us with two possibilities: either Brownson is Brown because he is possessed of Brown's brain, or he is Brown because he is psychologically continuous with Brown.

To decide between these alternatives, let us carry our thought experiment further still. Many people have survived with half their brain destroyed. Let us imagine that Brownson's brain (or indeed anyone's brain, say, Smith's brain) is now split into two equal halves or hemispheres, and that each hemisphere is inserted into a brainless body of its own. Following this operation, two men awake who share the same traits and memories as Smith, and who can both be said to be psychologically continuous with Smith. Are these men both Smith? And if so, are they also each other? Most people would argue that, even though the two men are very similar, they are in fact two different people.

So what can we conclude from this mind-boggling discussion, and what are the implications for personality? It seems that what makes you a person, what makes you 'a self-conscious mental being', depends causally upon the existence of your brain, but at the same time amounts to something more than just your brain. What this might be is unclear, and perhaps for a reason. As human beings, we have a tendency to think of our personhood as something concrete and tangible, something that exists 'out there' and extends through space and time. However, it is possible that personhood is nothing but a product of our minds, merely a convenient concept or schema that enables us to relate our present self with our past, future, and conditional selves, and, in so doing, to create an illusion of coherence and continuity from a jumble of disparate experiences.

If this is so, it need not be terminal for our definition of personality, which was rendered as 'a person's pattern of thinking, feeling, and behaving'. Nevertheless, if our concept of personality relies on our concept of personhood, then it probably shares the same ontological status (form of being) as personhood. This suggests that personality is a patterning principle, or set of patterning principles, and that threats to the pattern are also threats to the self, leading to distortion in the form of self-deception, or disintegration in the form of mental disorder.

Holding this in mind, let us turn to the problem of free will. Personality is born out of both genetic and environmental factors such as expectations regarding gender role and other social and cultural expectations that shape and constrain it. It is generally acquired or 'fixed' in childhood and adolescence, and does not change much thereafter, although certain aspects may change in small increments as a person acquires greater experience and understanding, including self-understanding.

If a person's personality is determined by genetic factors that he cannot change, environmental factors that he is born into and has no control over, and even freak accidents such as that suffered by Phineas Gage, then to what extent can he be held responsible for who he is? And if he cannot be held responsible for who he is, then to what extent can he be held responsible for what he does?

If he goes on to commit a serious crime, his criminal conviction depends on evidence proving beyond reasonable doubt that he carried out the act (*actus reus*) and *deliberately* intended or risked a harmful outcome (*mens rea*). However, 'insanity' at the time of the offence can be offered in his defence. According to the McNaghten rules prevalent in England and Wales, a plea to insanity can be made if it can be demonstrated that a person was suffering from a mental disorder at the time of the offence, and that this mental disorder led to an absence of *mens rea*. If the jurors decide on the balance of probabilities to accept this defence, the accused is found 'not guilty by reason of insanity'.

This gives rise to an important question: where should jurors draw the line between sanity and insanity? In allowing that a person with a mental disorder might not act deliberately or freely, the law is presupposing that people do ordinarily act freely, and, therefore, that free will exists. But is anyone ever capable of acting freely?*

The so-called problem of free will has long exercised the greatest minds, and has been tagged as the most important and pressing problem in all philosophy. Although the future may seem full of possibilities, many thinkers have argued that there can only be one possible future, one single way for things to unfold and pan out.

When Barack Obama became US President in January 2009, this fact was already true 2,000 years ago. Similarly, if he goes on to

---

*   An argument could be made that the criminal justice system exists not to punish wrongdoers but to maintain social order. If sentencing rests on social consequences rather than individual intentions, the existence or non-existence of free will becomes somewhat moot.

become UN Secretary General, this fact was already true 2,000 years ago, and is also true today, even though we cannot as yet know that it is true.

The so-called 'timelessness of truth' might lead us to conclude that the future has been pre-determined, and thus that we have no meaningful control over our actions. Thankfully, this sort of thinking is misguided. Although it was true 2,000 years ago, the fact that Obama became US President in January 2009 was not a fact about 2,000 years ago, but a fact about January 2009. It was true 2,000 years ago *because* Obama became US President in January 2009, not *vice versa*.

If the future is predetermined, it cannot be changed by anything that we might do. The standard form of this fatalist argument was popular in London during the Blitz. Either you are going to be killed by a bomb or you are not going to be killed by a bomb: if you are going to be killed by a bomb, any precautions you take will be futile; if you are not going to be killed by a bomb, any precautions you take will be superfluous.

Like the previous argument featuring Obama, this argument is flawed. The fact that you are not going to be killed by a bomb does not imply that you are not going to be killed by a bomb even if you do not take any precautions. It could be that you are not going to be killed by a bomb precisely because you did take some precautions. Imagine that you fall off your bicycle and hit your head, but, owing to the helmet that you are wearing, do not suffer any serious injuries. It would be churlish to argue that, because you did not suffer any serious injuries, you might as well not have been wearing a helmet.

Although the threat posed to free will by the timelessness of truth seems to have been dealt with, there is another sense in which there is only one possible future, one unique way for things to unfold and pan out. Given the physical state of the universe at any given point in time, and given the laws of physics which are universal and constant, (a) it is impossible for the history of the universe to be any other than it is, and (b) it is at least theoretically possible to map out every single past and future event in the universe. Hence, all past and future events are contained in the very fabric of the universe.

Some 200 years ago, the Marquis de Laplace transmogrified this concept of 'causal determinism' into a super-intelligent daemon who could accurately predict the future, first, by knowing every single physical fact about the universe, and, second, by applying Newton's Laws to those facts.

Of course, Newtonian physics has since been superseded by quantum mechanics, which allows for chance, or indeterminism, in the behaviour of elementary particles. Even so, quantum mechanics has not put paid to traditional concerns about causal determinism because (1) even if quantum mechanics is not one day to be replaced by a more comprehensive deterministic theory, indeterminism in the behaviour of elementary particles need not translate into indeterminism in human behaviour, and, (2) even if it did, the human behaviour that resulted would be random and unpredictable rather than free and responsible.

In short, while free will appears to be incompatible with determinism, it also appears to be incompatible with indeterminism!

Assuming that the deterministic view is broadly correct, is it still possible to argue in favour of free will? Philosopher Harry Frankfurt (born 1929) tried to do just that through the following thought experiment. Suppose that Smith forms the intention to rob a bank, devises a cunning plan, and carries it out successfully. Unbeknown to Smith, an evil daemon had been monitoring his brain, and had been prepared to intervene had Smith shown any signs of hesitation in executing his plan. Had Smith wanted to change his mind, he would not have been able to do so. However, Smith had not wanted to change his mind, and, in that much, he acted out of his own free will.

Frankfurt's thought experiment shows that free will is not incompatible with the inability to do otherwise—in other words, that it is not incompatible with determinism.

While Frankfurt's reasoning is no doubt correct, his idea of free will is a far cry from yours or mine. For most people, free will involves not only the ability to do something, but also the ability to do otherwise. When we talk of free will or freedom, we do not just mean 'unconstrained choice', but also control over that choice.

Philosopher Galen Strawson (born 1952) has argued that the very notion of free will—the one held by you and me—is simply incoherent. Self-determination requires us to be morally responsible for what we do. To be morally responsible for what we do, we need to be responsible for our mental nature. But that, as we have seen, is simply impossible. If you still think that you can be responsible for your mental nature, consider this: to be responsible for your mental nature, you need a prior mental nature, and to be responsible for that prior mental nature, you need a still prior mental nature, and so on *ad infinitum*. Thus, like personhood, free will may be nothing more than a product of our minds, nothing but a means of creating meaning out of meaninglessness.

16

Nothwithstanding these reservations about personhood and free will, let us open the discussion on personality disorders.

The study of human personality or 'character' (from the Greek *charaktêr*, the mark impressed upon a coin) dates back at least to antiquity. In his *Characters*, Tyrtamus (371-287 BC)—nicknamed Theophrastus or 'divinely speaking' by his contemporary Aristotle— divided the people of the Athens of the 4th century BC into thirty different personality types (Table 1.1). The *Characters* exerted a strong influence on subsequent studies of human personality such as those of Thomas Overbury (1581-1613) in England and Jean de la Bruyère (1645-1696) in France.

Table 1.1: Theophrastus' 30 character types			
Flattery	Unseasonableness	Grossness	Meanness
Complaisance	Officiousness	Garrulity	Avarice
Surliness	Unpleasantness	Loquacity	Cowardice
Arrogance	Offensiveness	Newsmaking	Superstition
Irony	Stupidity	Evil-speaking	Patronage of rascals
Boastfulness	Boorishness	Grumbling	
Petty ambition	Shamelessness	Distrustfulness	The aristocratic temper

The concept of personality disorder itself is much more recent and tentatively dates back to psychiatrist Philippe Pinel's 1801 description of *manie sans délire*, a condition which he character- ized as outbursts of rage and violence (*manie*) in the absence of any symptoms of psychosis such as delusions and hallucinations (*délires*).

Across the English Channel, physician JC Prichard (1786-1848) coined the term 'moral insanity' in 1835 to refer to a larger group of people characterized by 'morbid perversion of the natural feelings, affections, inclinations, temper, habits, moral dispositions and natural impulses', but the term, probably considered too broad and non-specific, soon fell into disuse.

Some 60 years on, in 1896, psychiatrist Emil Kraepelin (1856-1926) described seven forms of antisocial behaviour under the umbrella of 'psychopathic personality', a term later broadened by Kraepelin's younger colleague Kurt Schneider (1887-1967) to include those who 'suffer from their abnormality'. Schneider's seminal volume of 1923, *Die psychopathischen Persönlichkeiten (Psychopathic Personalities)*, still forms the basis of current classifications of personality disorders such as that contained in the influential American classification of mental disorders, the Diagnostic and Statistical Manual of Mental Disorders 5th Revision (DSM-5).

According to DSM-5, a personality disorder can be diagnosed if there are significant impairments in self and interpersonal functioning together with one or more pathological personality traits. In addition, these features must be (1) relatively stable across time and consistent across situations, (2) not better understood as normative for the individual's developmental stage or social and cultural environment, and (3) not solely due to the direct effects of a substance or general medical condition.

DSM-5 lists ten personality disorders, and allocates each to one of three groups or 'clusters': A, B, or C (Table 1.2).

Table 1.2: DSM-IV classification of personality disorders		
Cluster	**Description**	**Personality disorders in the cluster**
A	Odd, bizarre, eccentric	Paranoid Schizoid Schizotypal
B	Dramatic, erratic	Antisocial Borderline Histrionic Narcissistic
C	Anxious, fearful	Avoidant Dependent Obsessive–compulsive (Anankastic)

Before going on to characterize these ten personality disorders, it should be emphasized that they are more the product of historical observation than of scientific study, and thus that they are rather vague and imprecise constructs. As a result, they rarely present in their classic 'textbook' form, but instead tend to blur into one another. Their division into three clusters in DSM-5 is intended to reflect this tendency, with any given personality disorder most likely to blur with other personality disorders within its cluster. For instance, in cluster A, paranoid personality is most likely to blur with schizoid personality disorder and schizotypal personality disorder (Table 1.2).

The majority of people with a personality disorder never come into contact with mental health services, and those who do usually do so in the context of another mental disorder or at a time of crisis, commonly after self-harming or breaking the law. Nevertheless, personality disorders are important to health professionals because they predispose to mental disorder, and affect the presentation and management of existing mental disorder. They also result in considerable distress and impairment, and so may need to be treated 'in their own right'. Whether this ought to be the remit of the health professions is a matter of debate and controversy, especially with regard to those personality disorders which predispose to criminal activity, and which are often treated with the primary purpose of preventing crime.

Cluster A comprises paranoid, schizoid, and schizotypal personality disorders.

Paranoid personality disorder (PD) is characterized by a pervasive distrust of others, including even friends, family, and partner. As a result, the person is guarded and suspicious, and constantly on the lookout for clues or suggestions to validate his fears. He also has a strong sense of personal rights: he is overly sensitive to setbacks and rebuffs, easily feels shame and humiliation, and persistently bears grudges. Unsurprisingly, he tends to withdraw from others and to struggle with building close relationships. The principal ego defence in paranoid PD is projection, which involves attributing one's unacceptable thoughts and feelings to other people (see later). A large long-term twin study found that paranoid PD is modestly heritable, and that it shares a portion of its genetic and environmental risk factors with schizoid PD and schizotypal PD.

The term 'schizoid' designates a natural tendency to direct attention toward one's inner life and away from the external world. A person with schizoid PD is detached and aloof and prone to introspection and fantasy. He has no desire for social or sexual relationships, is indifferent to others and to social norms and conventions, and lacks emotional response. A competing theory about people with schizoid PD is that they are in fact highly sensitive with a rich inner life: they experience a deep longing for intimacy but find initiating and maintaining close relationships too difficult or distressing, and so retreat into their inner world. People with schizoid PD rarely present to medical attention because, despite their reluctance to form close relationships, they are generally well functioning, and quite untroubled by their apparent oddness.

Schizotypal PD is characterized by oddities of appearance, behaviour, and speech, unusual perceptual experiences, and anomalies of thinking similar to those seen in schizophrenia. These latter can include odd beliefs, magical thinking (for instance, thinking that speaking of the devil can make him appear), suspiciousness, and obsessive ruminations. People with schizotypal PD often fear social interaction and think of others as harmful. This may lead them to develop so-called ideas of reference, that is, beliefs or intuitions that events and happenings are somehow related to them. So whereas people with schizotypal PD and people with schizoid PD both avoid social interaction, with the former it is because they fear others, whereas with the latter it is because they have no desire to interact with others or find interacting with others too difficult. People with schizotypal PD have a higher than average probability of developing schizophrenia, and, indeed, the condition used to be called 'latent schizophrenia'.

Cluster B comprises antisocial, borderline, histrionic, and narcissistic personality disorders.

Until psychiatrist Kurt Schneider broadened the concept of personality disorder to include those who 'suffer from their abnormality', personality disorder was more or less synonymous with antisocial personality disorder. Antisocial PD is much more common in men than in women, and is characterized by a callous unconcern for the feelings of others. The person disregards social rules and obligations, is irritable and aggressive, acts impulsively, lacks guilt, and fails to learn from experience. In many cases, he has no difficulty finding relationships—and can even appear superficially charming (the so-called 'charming psychopath')—but these relationships are usually fiery, turbulent, and short-lived. As antisocial PD is the mental disorder most closely correlated with crime, he is likely to have a criminal record or a history of being in and out of prison.

Although a personality disorder cannot be diagnosed before adulthood, the presence of three types of behaviour in children—sometimes referred to as Macdonald's triad—is thought to predict the later development of antisocial PD: bedwetting, cruelty to animals, and pyromania (impulsive fire-setting for gratification or relief). A proportion of people with antisocial PD also meet the criteria for psychopathy, which is a similar but narrower construct.

In borderline PD (or emotionally unstable PD), the person essentially lacks a sense of self, and, as a result, experiences feelings of emptiness and fears of abandonment. There is a pattern of intense but unstable relationships, emotional instability, outbursts of anger and violence (especially in response to criticism), and impulsive behaviour. Suicidal threats and acts of self-harm are common, for which reason many people with borderline PD frequently come to medical attention. Borderline PD was so called because it was thought to lie on the 'borderline' between neurotic (anxiety) disorders and psychotic disorders such as schizophrenia and bipolar disorder.

It has been suggested that borderline personality disorder often results from childhood sexual abuse, and that it is more common in women in part because women are more likely to suffer sexual abuse. However, feminists have argued that borderline PD is more common in women because women presenting with angry and promiscuous behaviour tend to be labelled with it, whereas men presenting with similar behaviour tend instead to be labelled with antisocial PD.

What follows is a typical case of borderline PD as seen through the lens of an emergency doctor:

> *Twenty-eight-year-old Miss GL was brought to A&E after taking an impulsive overdose. The overdose was prompted by an argument with her boyfriend, Jack, during which he threatened to end their relationship. Jack reported that Miss GL took an overdose of 16 paracetamol tablets just as he had his foot in the front door. As she swallowed the tablets, she screamed out, 'I hate you! Look at me, I'm going to die and it's all your fault!' Medical records reveal that Miss GL last took an overdose only three months ago, in the heat of an argument with her mother. They also reveal that she has used all kinds of drugs, and that she had a road traffic accident only nine months ago. Furthermore, she has dropped out of two college courses and has never held down a job for more than six months. By the time she left A&E, Miss GL was no longer angry but excited at the prospect of going out for a meal with Jack.*

People with histrionic PD lack a sense of self-worth, and depend for their wellbeing on attracting the attention and approval of others. They often seem to be dramatizing or 'playing a part' in a bid to be heard and seen. Indeed, 'histrionic' derives from the

Latin *histrionicus*, 'pertaining to the actor'. People with histrionic PD may take great care of their appearance and behave in a manner that is overly charming or inappropriately seductive. As they crave excitement and act on impulse or suggestion, they can place them-selves at risk of accident or exploitation. Their dealings with others often seem insincere or superficial, which, in the longer term, can adversely impact on their social and romantic relationships. This is especially distressing to them, as they are sensitive to criticism and rejection, and react badly to loss or failure. A vicious circle may take hold in which the more rejected they feel, the more histrionic they become; and the more histrionic they become, the more rejected they feel. It can be argued that a vicious circle of some kind is at the heart of every personality disorder, and, indeed, every mental disorder.

In narcissistic PD, the person has an excessively high regard for his own importance, a sense of entitlement, and a need to be admired. He is envious of others and expects them to be the same of him. He lacks empathy and readily exploits others to achieve his aims. To others, he may seem self-absorbed, controlling, intolerant, selfish, or insensitive. If he feels obstructed or ridiculed, he can fly into a fit of destructive anger and revenge. Such a reaction is sometimes called 'narcissistic rage', and can have disastrous consequences for all those involved.

Narcissistic personality disorder is named for the Greek myth of Narcissus, of which there are several versions. In Ovid's version, which is the most commonly related, the nymph Echo falls in love with Narcissus, a youth of extraordinary beauty. As a child, Narcissus had been prophesized by Teiresias, the blind prophet of Thebes, to 'live to a ripe old age, as long as he never knows himself'.

One day, Echo followed Narcissus through the woods as he went about hunting for stags. She longed to speak to him but dared not utter the first word. Overhearing her footsteps, the youth cried out, 'Who's there?' to which she responded, 'Who's there?' When at last she revealed herself, she rushed out to embrace Narcissus, but he scorned her and pushed her away. Echo spent the rest of her life pining for Narcissus, and slowly withered away until there was nothing left of her but her voice. Then one day, Narcissus went to quench his thirst at a pool of water. Seeing his own image in the water, he fell in love with it. But each time he bent down to kiss it, it seemed to disappear. Narcissus grew ever more thirsty, but would not leave or disturb the pool of water for fear of losing sight of his reflection. In the end, he died of thirst, and there, on that very spot, appeared the narcissus flower, with its bright face and bowed neck.

Cluster C comprises avoidant, dependent, and anankastic personality disorders.

People with avoidant PD believe that they are socially inept, unappealing, or inferior, and constantly fear being embarrassed, criticized, or rejected. They avoid meeting others unless they are certain of being liked, and are restrained even in their intimate relationships. Avoidant PD is strongly associated with anxiety disorders, and may also be associated with actual or felt rejection by parents or peers in childhood. Research suggests that people with avoidant PD excessively monitor internal reactions, both their own and those of others, which prevents them from engaging naturally or fluently in social situations. A vicious circle takes hold in which the more they monitor their internal reactions, the more inept they feel; and the more inept they feel, the more they monitor their internal reactions. Self-oblivion is often all that is required to carry the day.

Dependent PD is characterized by a lack of self-confidence and an excessive need to be looked after. The person needs a lot of help in making everyday decisions and surrenders important life decisions to the care of others. He greatly fears abandonment and may go through considerable lengths to secure and maintain relationships. A person with dependent PD sees himself as inadequate and helpless, and so surrenders personal responsibility and submits himself to one or more protective others. He imagines that he is at one with these protective other(s), whom he idealizes as competent and powerful, and towards whom he behaves in a manner that is ingratiating and self-effacing. People with dependent PD often pair up with people with a cluster B personality disorder, who feed on the unconditional high regard in which they are held. Overall, people with dependent PD maintain a naïve and child-like perspective, and have limited insight into themselves and others. This entrenches their dependency, and leaves them vulnerable to abuse and exploitation.

Anankastic PD is characterized by excessive preoccupation with details, rules, lists, order, organization, or schedules; perfectionism so extreme that it prevents a task from being completed; and devotion to work and productivity at the expense of leisure and relationships. A person with anankastic PD is typically doubting and cautious, rigid and controlling, humorless, and miserly. His underlying anxiety arises from a perceived lack of control over a world that eludes his understanding; and the more he tries to exert control, the more out of control he feels. In consequence, he has little tolerance for complexity or nuance, and tends to simplify the world by seeing things as either all good or all bad. His relationships with colleagues, friends, and family are often strained by the rigid and unreasonable demands that he makes upon them.

People with anankastic PD tend to view their obsessions as rational and consistent with their self-image ('egosyntonic'), whereas people with obsessive-compulsive disorder tend to view their obsessions as irrational and inconsistent with their self-image ('egodystonic').

While personality disorders may differ from mental disorders like schizophrenia and bipolar disorder, they do, by definition, lead to significant impairment. They are estimated to affect about 10 per cent of people, although this figure ultimately depends on where clinicians draw the line between a 'normal' personality and one that leads to significant impairment. Characterizing the ten personality disorders is difficult, but diagnosing them reliably is even more so. For instance, how far from the norm must personality traits deviate before they can be counted as disordered? How significant is 'significant impairment'? And how is 'impairment' to be defined?

Whatever the answers to these questions, they are bound to include a large part of subjectivity. Personal dislike, prejudice, or a clash of values can all play a part in arriving at a diagnosis of personality disorder, and it has been argued that the diagnosis amounts to little more than a convenient label for undesirables and social deviants.

While personality disorders may lead to 'severe impairment', they may also lead to extraordinary achievement. A 2005 study by Board and Fritzon found that histrionic, narcissistic, and anankastic personality disorders are *more* common in high-level executives than in mentally disordered criminal offenders at the high security Broadmoor Hospital.

This suggests that people often benefit from non-normative and potentially maladaptive personality traits. For instance, people with histrionic personality disorder may be more adept at charming and cajoling others, and therefore at building and exercising professional relationships. People with narcissistic personality disorder may be highly ambitious, confident, and self-motivated, and able to employ people and situations to maximum advantage. And people with anankastic personality disorder may get quite far up their career ladder simply by being so devoted to work and productivity. Even people with borderline personality disorder may at times be bright, witty, and the life and soul of the party.

In their study, Board and Fritzon described the executives with a personality disorder as 'successful psychopaths' and the criminal offenders as 'unsuccessful psychopaths', and it may be that highly successful people and disturbed psychopaths have more in common than first meets the eye. As psychologist and philosopher William James (1842-1910) put it, 'When a superior intellect and a psychopathic temperament coalesce… in the same individual, we have the best possible condition for the kind of effective genius that gets into the biographical dictionaries.'

More recently, in 2010, Mullins-Sweatt and her colleagues carried out a study to uncover how successful psychopaths differ from unsuccessful ones. They asked a number of members of Division 41 (psychology and law) of the American Psychological Association, professors of clinical psychology, and criminal attorneys to first identify, and then to rate and describe, one of their acquaintances (if any) who could be counted as successful and who also conformed to psychologist Robert Hare's definition of a psychopath:

> …*social predators who charm, manipulate and ruthlessly plow their way through life … Completely lacking in conscience and feeling for others, they selfishly take what they want and do as they please, violating social norms and expectations without the slightest sense of guilt or regret.*

From the responses they collated, Mullins-Sweatt and her team found that successful psychopaths matched unsuccessful ones in all respects but one, namely, conscientiousness. So it seems that the key difference between unsuccessful and successful psychopaths is that the former behave impulsively and irresponsibly, whereas the latter are able to inhibit or restrain those destructive tendencies and build for the future.

Intelligence and conscientiousness are not enough to guarantee success, which also requires traits such as ambition, motivation, and people skills—traits that may be particularly pronounced when rooted in a personality disorder.

Personality disorders are generally thought to arise from a combination of genetic factors and traumatic early life experiences such as parental loss and emotional, physical, and sexual abuse. People who have suffered childhood trauma may be left with intense feelings of despair, helplessness, and worthlessness. Later in life, they may seek out achievement and success to help compensate for these feelings. For instance, they may wish to be recognized by strangers because they were not recognized by their own parents, or they may wish to have control over others because they had none when they needed it most. The drive for achievement and success combined with the character traits and resilience that arise from loss and trauma may in later life propel them to the highest echelons of society.

This is borne out by a large study that looked at almost 700 eminent personalities, and found that 45 per cent had lost a parent before the age of 21. This 'orphanhood effect' seems particularly marked in creative people. One study looking specifically at a sample of authors found that 55 per cent had lost a parent before the age of 15.

This suggests that disturbed psychopaths and creative visionaries do indeed share many features. While the former suffer from them, the latter are (also) able to put them to good use.

Broadly speaking, anyone's personality can be said to lead to distress and impairment. For instance, a gregarious student is unable to isolate himself in the library and ends up failing his exams. A zealous company director loses his temper and regrets the damage that he has done to himself, others, and his company. An upstanding whistleblower ends up losing his job.

Everyone suffers for who he is, and, very often, our greatest strength is also the germ of our deepest suffering. While it is impossible to avoid such suffering, it is at least possible to value it for the personal growth that it can bring.

Like many blind figures in classical mythology, the prophet Teiresias could 'see' into himself. This self-knowledge enabled him not only to understand himself, but also to understand others and so to 'see into the future'. Similarly, our suffering prompts us to look into ourselves. The self-knowledge this brings enables us not only to better regulate ourselves, but also to better appreciate others, the world, and our place within it. Thus, our suffering transforms our lives into a journey, a journey without an end, perhaps, but one that can also be seen as an end-in-itself. It is in this way that our suffering, or 'impairment', can bring deep meaning to our lives.

What if your personality did not lead you to suffer? What, in other words, if you had an 'ideal' personality? In the *Nicomachean Ethics*, Aristotle remarks on human conduct that, 'Men may be bad in many ways, but good in one way only.' If there could be an ideal personality, there could only be one such personality, and anyone with an ideal personality would have the same personality.

A person with an ideal personality would in some sense be god-like, and, like God, impossible to imagine or define, and impossible to improve upon. Conversely, people with a personality disorder have great scope for self-improvement, or, in the words of Aristotle, for the 'refinement of virtue and judgement'. Returning to the journey metaphor, they are able to embark on a much longer, more varied, and more eventful journey, and, armed with their heart-rending experiences and hard-won wisdom, may arrive much further in the end. The most fulfilling novels and stories are invariably those in which the hero develops his character through renewed trials and tribulations. Without these obstacles, there would be no journey, no story, and no life.

In Freudian psychoanalytic theory, ego defences are unconscious processes that we deploy to diffuse the fear and anxiety that arise when who we think we are or who we think we should be (our conscious 'superego') comes into conflict with who we really are (our unconscious 'id').

For instance, at an unconscious level a man may find himself attracted to another man, but at a conscious level he may find this attraction flatly unacceptable. To diffuse the anxiety that arises from this conflict, he may deploy one or several ego defences. For example, (1) he might refuse to admit to himself that he is attracted to this man. Or (2) he might superficially adopt ideas and behaviours that are diametrically opposed to those of a stereotypical homosexual, such as going out for several pints with the lads, banging his fists on the counter, and peppering his speech with loud profanities. Or (3) he might transfer his attraction onto someone else and then berate *him* for being gay (young children can teach us much through playground retorts such as 'mirror, mirror' and 'what you say is what you are'). In each case, the man has used a common ego defence, respectively, repression, reaction formation, and projection.

Repression can be thought of as 'motivated forgetting': the active, albeit unconscious, 'forgetting' of unacceptable drives, emotions, ideas, or memories. Repression is often confused with denial, which is the refusal to admit to certain unacceptable or unmanageable aspects of reality. Whereas repression relates to mental or internal stimuli, denial relates to external stimuli. That said, repression and denial often work together, and can be difficult to disentangle.

Repression can also be confused with distortion, which is the reshaping of reality to suit one's inner needs. For instance, a person who has been beaten black and blue by his father no longer recalls these traumatic events (repression), and instead sees his father as a gentle and loving man (distortion). In this example, there is a clear sense of the distortion not only building upon but also reinforcing the repression.

Reaction formation is the superficial adoption—and, often, exag-geration—of emotions and impulses that are diametrically opposed to one's own. A possible high-profile case of reaction formation is that of a particular US congressman, who, as chairman of the Missing and Exploited Children's Caucus, introduced legislation to protect children from exploitation by adults over the Internet. The congressman resigned when it later emerged that he had been exchanging sexually explicit electronic messages with a teenage boy. Other, classic, examples of reaction formation include the alcoholic who extolls the virtues of abstinence and the rich student who attends and even organizes anti-capitalist rallies.

Projection is the attribution of one's unacceptable thoughts and feelings to others. Like distortion, projection necessarily involves repression as a first step, since unacceptable thoughts and feelings need to be repudiated before they can be attributed to others. Classic examples of projection include the envious person who believes that everyone envies him, the covetous person who lives in constant fear of being dispossessed, and the person with fantasies of infidelity who suspects that his partner is cheating on him.

As aforementioned, people with anankastic personality disorder tend to simplify the world by seeing things as either all good or all bad. This ego defence, called splitting, is very common, and can be defined as the division or polarization of beliefs, actions, objects, or people into good and bad by selectively focusing on either their positive or negative attributes. This is often seen in politics, for instance, when left-wingers caricature right-wingers as selfish and narrow-minded, and right-wingers caricature left-wingers as irresponsible and self-serving hypocrites. Other classic examples of splitting are the religious zealot who divides people into blessed and damned, and the child of divorcees who idolizes one parent while shunning the other. Splitting diffuses the anxiety that arises from our inability to grasp a complex and nuanced state of affairs by simplifying and schematizing it so that it can more readily be processed or accepted.

Splitting also arises in groups, with people inside the group being seen in a positive light, and people outside the group in a negative light. Another phenomenon that occurs in groups is groupthink, which is not strictly speaking an ego defence, but which is so important as to be worthy of mention. Groupthink arises when members of a group unconsciously seek to minimize conflict by failing to critically test, analyse, and evaluate ideas. As a result, decisions reached by the group tend to be more irrational than those that would have been reached by any one member of the group acting alone. Even married couples can fall into groupthink, for instance, when they decide to take their holidays in places that neither wanted, but thought that the other wanted. Groupthink arises because members of a group are afraid both of criticizing and of being criticized, and also because of the hubristic sense of confidence and invulnerability that arises from being in a group. Philosopher Ludwig Wittgenstein (1889-1951) once remarked, 'It is a good thing that I did not let myself be influenced.' In a similar vein, historian Edward Gibbon (1737-1794) wrote that '…solitude is the school of genius … and the uniformity of a work denotes the hand of a single artist'. In short, a camel is a horse designed by a committee.

An ego defence similar to splitting is idealization. Like the positive end of splitting, idealization involves overestimating the positive attributes of a person, object, or idea while underestimating its negative attributes. More fundamentally, it involves the projection of our needs and desires onto that person, object, or idea. A paradigm of idealization is infatuation, when love is confused with the need to love, and the idealized person's negative attributes are glossed over or even imagined as positive. Although this can make for a rude awakening, there are few better ways of relieving our existential anxiety than by manufacturing something that is 'perfect' for us, be it a piece of equipment, a place, country, person, or god.

If in love with someone inaccessible, it might be more convenient to intellectualize our love, perhaps by thinking of it in terms of idealization! In intellectualization, uncomfortable feelings associated with a problem are repressed by thinking about the problem in cold and abstract terms. I once received a phone call from a junior doctor in psychiatry in which he described a recent in-patient admission as 'a 47-year-old mother of two *who attempted to cessate her life as a result of being diagnosed with a metastatic mitotic lesion*'. A formulation such as '…who tried to kill herself after being told that she is dying of cancer' would have been better English, but all too effective at evoking the full horror of this poor lady's predicament.

Intellectualization should not be confused with rationalization, which is the use of feeble but seemingly plausible arguments either to justify something that is painful to accept ('sour grapes') or to make it seem 'not so bad after all' ('sweet lemons'). For instance, a person who has been rejected by a love interest convinces himself that she rejected him because she did not share in his ideal of happiness (sour grapes), and also that her rejection is a blessing in disguise in that it has freed him to find a more suitable partner (sweet lemons).

While no one can altogether avoid deploying ego defences, some ego defences are thought to be more 'mature' than others, not only because they involve some degree of insight, but also because they can be adaptive or useful. If a person is angry at his boss, he may go home and kick the dog, or he may instead go out and play a good game of tennis. The first instance (kicking the dog) is an example of displacement, the redirection of uncomfortable feelings towards someone or something less important, which is an immature ego defence. The second instance (playing a good game of tennis) is an example of sublimation, the channelling of uncomfortable feelings into socially condoned and often productive activities, which is a much more mature ego defence.

There are a number of mature ego defences like sublimation that can be substituted for the more primitive ones. Altruism, for instance, can in some cases be a form of sublimation in which a person copes with his anxiety by stepping outside himself and helping others. By concentrating on the needs of others, people in altruistic vocations such as medicine or teaching may be able to permanently push their own needs into the background. Conversely, people who care for a disabled or elderly person may experience profound anxiety and distress when this role is suddenly removed from them.

Another mature ego defence is humour. By seeing the absurd or ridiculous aspect of an emotion, event, or situation, a person is able to put it into a less threatening context and thereby diffuse the anxiety that it gives rise to. In addition, he is able to share, and test, his insight with others in the benign and gratifying form of a joke. If man laughs so much, it is no doubt because he has the most developed unconscious in the animal kingdom. The things that people laugh about most are their errors and inadequacies; the difficult challenges that they face around personal identity, social standing, sexual relationships, and death; and incongruity, absurdity, and meaninglessness. These are all deeply human concerns: just as no one has ever seen a laughing dog, so no one has ever heard of a laughing god.

Further up the maturity scale is asceticism, which is the denial of the importance of that which most people fear or strive for, and so of the very grounds for anxiety and disappointment. If fear is, ultimately, for oneself, then the denial of the self removes the very grounds for fear. People in modern societies are much more anxious than people in traditional or historical societies, no doubt because of the strong emphasis that modern societies place on the self as an independent and autonomous agent.

In the Hindu *Bhagavad Gita*, the god Krishna appears to Arjuna in the midst of the Battle of Kurukshetra, and advises him not to succumb to his scruples but to do his duty and fight on. In either case, all the men on the battlefield are one day condemned to die, as are all men. Their deaths are trivial, because the spirit in them, their human essence, does not depend on their particular incarnations for its continued existence. Krishna says, 'When one sees eternity in things that pass away and infinity in finite things, then one has pure knowledge.'

> *There has never been a time when you and I have not existed, nor will there be a time when we will cease to exist … the wise are not deluded by these changes.*

There are a great number of ego defences, and the combinations and circumstances in which we use them reflect on our personality. Indeed, one could go so far as to argue that the self is nothing but the sum of its ego defences, which are constantly shaping, upholding, protecting, and repairing it.

The self is like a cracked mask that is in constant need of being pieced together. But behind the mask there is nobody at home.

While we cannot entirely escape from ego defences, we can gain some insight into how we use them. This self-knowledge, if we have the courage for it, can awaken us to ourselves, to others, and to the world around us, and free us to express our full potential as human beings.

The greatest oracle of the ancient world was the oracle at Delphi, and inscribed on the forecourt of the temple of Apollo at Delphi was a simple two-word command:

Γνῶθι σεαυτόν
Know thyself.

Chapter 2

Schizophrenia, the price for being human

If you talk to God, you are praying. If God talks to you,
you have schizophrenia.

—Thomas Szasz

The term 'schizophrenia' was coined in 1910 by psychiatrist*
Paul Eugen Bleuler (1857-1939), and is derived from the
Greek words *schizo* ('split') and *phren* ('mind'). Although people often
mistakenly think of schizophrenia as a 'split personality', Bleuler had
intended the term to reflect the 'loosening' of thoughts and feelings
which he had found to be a prominent feature of the illness.

Robert Louis Stevenson's novel *The Strange Case of Dr Jekyll
and Mr Hyde* did much to popularize the concept of a 'split
personality', which is sometimes also referred to as 'multiple

---

* People often confuse psychiatrist, psychologist, psychotherapist, and psychoanalyst.
  A psychiatrist is a medical doctor specialized in the diagnosis and treatment of
  mental disorders such as schizophrenia and depression. A clinical psychologist is
  an expert in human experience and behaviour, and typically devotes a lot of time
  to understanding patients and their carers. A psychotherapist is any person trained
  in delivering specialized talking treatments, commonly a clinical psychologist or
  psychiatrist. Finally, a psychoanalyst is a type of psychotherapist trained in delivering
  specialized talking treatments based on the psychoanalytic principles pioneered by
  Sigmund Freud and others.

personality disorder'. However, multiple personality disorder is a vanishingly rare condition that is entirely unrelated to schizophrenia. The vast majority of psychiatrists have never seen a case of multiple personality disorder, and many think that the condition does not even exist. Although schizophrenia sufferers may hear voices that they attribute to various entities, or harbour strange beliefs that seem out of keeping with their usual selves, this is not the same as having a 'split personality'. Unlike Dr Jekyll, schizophrenia sufferers do not suddenly mutate into a different, unrecognizable person.

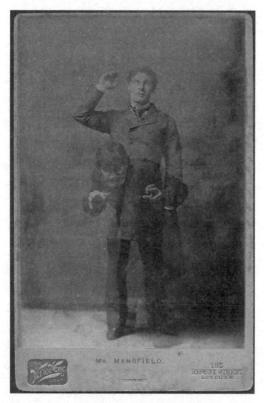

Figure 2.1. Double exposure photograph (1895) of Richard Mansfield, who played the roles of both Dr Jekyll and Mr Hyde.

Unfortunately, the term 'schizophrenia' has led to much confusion about the nature of the illness. Ironically, Bleuler had intended it to clarify matters by replacing the older, even more misleading term of *dementia praecox* ('dementia of early life'). This older term had been championed by Emil Kraepelin, who wrongly believed that the illness only occurred in young people and inevitably led to mental deterioration. Bleuler disagreed on both counts, and so renamed the illness 'schizophrenia'. He held that, contrary to mental deterioration, schizophrenia led to a sharpening of the senses and to a heightened consciousness of memories and experiences.

It is as common as it is unfortunate to hear the adjective 'schizophrenic' being bandied about to mean 'changeable', 'volatile', or 'unpredictable'. This usage, which ought to be discouraged, perpetuates people's misunderstanding of the illness and contributes to the stigmatization of schizophrenia sufferers. Even used correctly, the term 'schizophrenic' does little more than label a person by an illness, implicitly diminishing him to little more than that illness. A person is not a 'schizophrenic' any more than he is a 'diabetic' or suffering with toothache.

Although Kraepelin had some misguided beliefs about the illness, he was he first person to distinguish it from other forms of psychosis, and in particular from the 'affective psychoses' that occur in mood disorders such as depression and bipolar disorder. His classification of mental disorders, the *Compendium der Psychiatrie*, is the forerunner of the two most influential classifications of mental disorders, the Diagnostic and Statistical Manual of Mental Disorders 5th Revision (DSM-5) and the International Classification of Diseases 10th Revision (ICD-10). As well as listing mental disorders, these classifications provide operational definitions and diagnostic criteria that physicians and researchers use in establishing or verifying diagnoses.

Kraepelin first isolated schizophrenia from other forms of psychosis in 1887, but that is not to say that schizophrenia—or *dementia praecox*, as he called it—had not existed long before his day. The oldest available description of an illness closely resembling schizophrenia can be found in the Ebers papyrus, which dates back to the Egypt of 1550 BC. And archaeological discoveries of Stone Age skulls with burr holes—drilled, presumably, to release evil spirits—have led to speculation that schizophrenia is as old as mankind itself.

In antiquity, people did not think of 'madness' (a term that they used indiscriminately for all forms of psychosis) in terms of mental disorder but of divine punishment or demonic possession. Evidence for this comes from the Old Testament, and more particularly the First Book of Samuel, which relates how King Saul became 'mad' after neglecting his religious duties and angering God. That David played on his harp to make Saul feel better suggests that, even in antiquity, people believed that psychotic disorders, or psychosis, could be successfully treated.

> *But the Spirit of the Lord departed from Saul, and an evil spirit from the Lord troubled him. And it came to pass, when the evil spirit from God was upon Saul, that David took an harp, and played with his hand: so Saul was refreshed, and was well, and the evil spirit departed from him.*

—1 Samuel 16:14, 23 (KJV)

In Greek mythology and the Homerian epics, madness is similarly thought of as a punishment from God—or the gods. Thus, Hera punished Herakles by 'sending madness upon him', and Agamemnon confided to Achilles that 'Zeus robbed me of my wits'. It is in fact not until the time of Hippocrates (460-377 BC) that madness first became an object of scientific speculation. Hippocrates thought that madness resulted from an imbalance of four bodily fluids or humours. Melancholy, for instance, resulted from an excess of black bile, and could be cured by restoring the balance of the bodily humours by such treatments as special diets, purgatives, and blood-lettings. To modern readers, Hippocrates' ideas may seem far-fetched, perhaps even on the dangerous side of eccentric, but in the 4th century BC they represented a significant advance on the idea of madness as divine punishment or demonic possession. Aristotle (384-322 BC) and, later, the Roman physician Galen (129-200) elaborated on Hippocrates' humoural theories, and both men played an important role in establishing them as Europe's dominant medical model.

Only from the brain springs our pleasures, our feelings of happiness, laughter and jokes, our pain, our sorrows and tears … This same organ makes us mad or confused, inspires us with fear and anxiety…

—Hippocrates, *The Holy Disease*

In Ancient Rome, physician Asclepiades (124-40 BC) and philosopher Cicero (106-43 BC) rejected Hippocrates' humoural theories, asserting, for example, that melancholy results not from an excess of black bile but from emotions such as grief, fear, and rage. Unfortunately, the influence of these luminaries began to decline in the 1st century AD, and physician Celsus (25 BC-50) reinstated the idea of madness as divine punishment or demonic possession, an idea which gained currency with the rise of Christianity and the decline of the Roman Empire.

In the Middle Ages, religion became central to cure, and, alongside the mediaeval asylums such as the Bethlehem (an infamous asylum in London that is at the origin of the expression, 'like a bad day at Bedlam'), some monasteries transformed themselves into centres for the treatment of mental disorder. This is not to say that the humoural theories of Hippocrates had been supplanted, but merely that they had been incorporated into the prevailing Christian dogma, with older treatments such as purgatives and blood-lettings continuing alongside the prayers and confession.

During the Middle Ages, classical ideas had been kept alive in Islamic centres such as Baghdad and Damascus, and their re-introduction by St Thomas Aquinas (1225-1274) and others in the 13th century once again led to an increased separation of mind and soul, and to a shift from the Platonic metaphysics of Christianity to the Aristotelian empiricism of science. This movement laid the foundations for the Renaissance, and, later, for the Enlightenment.

The burning of the so-called heretics, often people suffering from psychotic disorders such as schizophrenia, began in the early Renaissance and reached its peak in the 14th and 15th centuries. First published in 1563, *De praestigiis daemonum (The Deception of Demons)* argued that the madness of heretics resulted not from supernatural forces but from natural causes. The Church proscribed the book and accused its author, Johann Weyer, of being a sorcerer.

From the 15th century, scientific breakthroughs such as the heliocentric system of astronomer Galileo (1564-1642) began challenging the authority of the Church. Man, not God, became the focus of attention and study, and it is also around this time that anatomist Vesalius (1514-1564) published his landmark *De humani corporis fabrica libri septem (The Seven Books on the Structure of the Human Body)*.

Despite the scientific developments of the Renaissance, Hippocrates' humoural theories perdured into the 17th and 18th centuries, to be mocked by playwright Molière (1622-1673) in such works as *Le Malade imaginaire (The Imaginary Invalid)* and *Le Médecin malgré lui (The Doctor in Spite of Himself)*. Empirical thinkers such as John Locke (1632-1704) in England and Denis Diderot (1713-1784) in France challenged this *status quo* by arguing, in the same vein as Cicero, that the psyche arises from sensations to produce reason and emotions.

Also in France, the physician Philippe Pinel (1745-1826) began regarding mental disorder as the result of exposure to psychological and social stressors, and, to a lesser extent, of heredity and physiological damage. A landmark in the history of psychiatry, Pinel's *Traité Médico-philosophique sur l'aliénation mentale ou la manie (A Treatise on Insanity)* called for a more humane approach to the treatment of mental disorder. This 'moral treatment', as it had already been dubbed, included respect for the patient, a trusting and confiding doctor-patient relationship, decreased stimuli, routine activity and occupation, and the abandonment of old-fashioned Hippocratic treatments. At about the same time as Pinel in France, the Tukes (father and son) in England founded the York Retreat, the first centre 'for the humane care of the insane' in the British Isles.

In the 19th century, hopes of successful cures lead to the burgeoning of mental hospitals in North America, Britain, and many of the countries of continental Europe. Unlike the mediaeval asylums, these hospitals treated the 'insane poor' according to the principles of moral treatment. Like Pinel before him, Jean-Etienne-Dominique Esquirol, Pinel's student and successor at the Salpêtrière Hospital, attempted a classification of mental disorders, and his resulting *Des Maladies mentales...* (*Concerning Mental Illnesses*) is regarded as the first modern treatise on clinical psychiatry. Half a century later, Kraepelin carried out his landmark classification of mental disorders, the *Compendium der Psychiatrie*, in which he distinguished schizophrenia (or *dementia praecox*) from other forms of psychosis. Kraepelin further distinguished three clinical presentations of schizophrenia: (1) paranoia, dominated by delusions and hallucinations; (2) hebephrenia, dominated by inappropriate reactions and behaviours; and (3) catatonia, dominated by extreme agitation or immobility and odd mannerisms and posturing.

In the early 20th century, psychiatrist Karl Jaspers (1883-1969) brought the methods of phenomenology—the direct investigation and description of phenomena as consciously experienced—into the field of clinical psychiatry. This so-called descriptive psychopathology created a scientific basis for the practice of psychiatry, and emphasized that symptoms of mental disorder should be diagnosed according to their form rather than to their content. This means, for example, that a belief is a delusion not because it is deemed implausible by a person in a position of authority, but because it conforms to the definition of a delusion, that is, 'a strongly held belief that is not amenable to logic or persuasion and that is out of keeping with its holder's background or culture.'

Sigmund Freud (1856-1939) and his disciples influenced much of 20th century psychiatry, and by the second half of the century a majority of psychiatrists in the US (although not in the UK) believed that mental disorders such as schizophrenia resulted from unconscious conflicts originating in early childhood. As a director of the US National Institute of Mental Health put it, 'From 1945 to 1955, it was nearly impossible for a non-psychoanalyst to become a chairman of a department or professor of psychiatry.'

In the latter part of the 20th century, neuroimaging techniques, genetic studies, and pharmacological breakthroughs such as the first antipsychotic drug chlorpromazine completely reversed this psychoanalytical model of mental disorder, and prompted a return to a more biological, 'neo-Kraepelinian' model.

At present, schizophrenia is primarily seen as a biological disorder of the brain, although it is also recognized that psychological and social stressors can play important roles in triggering episodes of illness, and that different approaches to treatment should be seen not as competing but as complementary.

However, critics tend to deride this 'bio-psycho-social' model as little more than a 'bio-bio-bio' model, with psychiatrists reduced to mere diagnosticians and pill pushers. Many critics question the scientific evidence underpinning such a robust biological approach, and call for a radical rethink of mental disorders, not as detached disease processes that can be cut up into diagnostic labels, but as subjective and meaningful experiences grounded in both personal and larger sociocultural narratives.

Still today, many people with schizophrenia and their relatives, friends, and carers do not talk openly about the illness for fear of being misunderstood or stigmatized. This deplorable state of affairs can create the impression that the condition is very rare. It is in fact so common that most of us will know at least one person suffering with it. The lifetime prevalence of schizophrenia varies according to how the condition is defined, and is often quoted as 1 per cent.

Schizophrenia can present at any age, but is rare in childhood and early adolescence. Most cases are diagnosed in late adolescence or early adulthood.

Unlike depressive and anxiety disorders, which are more common in women, schizophrenia affects men and women in more or less equal numbers. However, it tends to present at a younger age in men, and to affect them more severely. Why this should be remains unclear.

Schizophrenia exists in all cultures and ethnic groups, but, surprisingly, tends to have more favourable outcomes in traditional societies. This may be because tight-knit communities are more tolerant of mental illness and more supportive of their mentally ill. If true, it suggests that interpretations and attitudes can exert an important influence on the outcome of the illness.

Generally speaking, schizophrenia is more common in inner cities and urban areas than in rural settings. This could be because the stress of urban living increases the risk of developing the illness (the 'breeder hypothesis'), or because people with the illness tend to gravitate to urban areas (the 'drift hypothesis').

The symptoms of schizophrenia are manifold, and present in such a variety of combinations and severities that it is impossible to describe a 'typical' case. In the short term, symptoms may wax and wane, with the sufferer experiencing both good days and bad days. In the longer term, the emphasis may shift from one group of symptoms to another, presenting different challenges for sufferer and carers.

The symptoms of schizophrenia are classically divided into three groups: positive symptoms, cognitive symptoms, and negative symptoms, as detailed in Table 2.1.

Table 2.1: Symptoms of schizophrenia	
Positive symptoms	Delusions Hallucinations } Psychotic symptoms
Cognitive symptoms	Difficulties with attention, concentration, and memory
Negative symptoms	Restricted amount and/or range of thought and speech Restricted range of emotions, or inappropriate emotions Loss of drive and motivation Social withdrawal

Positive symptoms consist of psychotic symptoms (hallucinations and delusions), which are usually as real to the sufferer as they are unreal to everyone else. Positive symptoms are considered to be the hallmark of schizophrenia, and tend to be most prominent in its early stages. They can be provoked or aggravated by stressful situations, such as leaving home for university, breaking off a relationship, or taking drugs (a form of biological, as opposed to psychological, stress).

Psychiatrists define a hallucination as 'a sense perception that arises in the absence of an external stimulus'. Hallucinations involve hearing, seeing, smelling, tasting, or feeling things that are not actually there. In schizophrenia, the most common hallucinations are auditory, involving voices and sounds. Voices can either speak *to* the sufferer (second-person—'you'—voices) or *about* him (third-person—'he'—voices). Voices can be highly distressing, especially if they involve threats or abuse, or if they are loud and incessant. One might begin to experience something of this distress by turning on the radio and the television, both at the same time and at full volume, and then attempting to hold a normal conversation. It should be noted that not all voices are distressing, and some, such as the voices of old acquaintances, dead ancestors, or guardian angels, can even be comforting or reassuring, and, at least in that much, may not be in need of 'curing'.

Delusions are defined as 'strongly held beliefs that are not amenable to logic or persuasion and that are out of keeping with their holder's background or culture'. Although delusions need not be false, the process by which they are arrived at is usually bizarre and illogical. In schizophrenia, delusions are most often of being persecuted or controlled, although they can also follow other themes. The most common delusional themes are listed in Table 2.2.

Table 2.2: Delusional themes in schizophrenia	
Delusions of persecution	Delusions of being persecuted – for example, being spied upon by secret services or being poisoned by aliens.
Delusions of control	Delusions that one's feelings, thoughts or actions are being controlled by an external force – for example, having one's thoughts 'stolen' by aliens and replaced by different thoughts.
Delusions of reference	Delusions that objects, events or other persons have a particular and unusual significance relating to oneself – for example, receiving a series of coded messages from the aliens while listening to a radio programme.

Delusions of grandeur	Delusions of being invested with special status, a special purpose or special abilities – for example, being the most intelligent person on earth and having the responsibility of saving it from climate change. Delusions of grandeur are more common in manic psychosis than in schizophrenia.
Religious delusions	Delusions of having a special relationship with God or a supernatural force, for example, being the next messiah or being persecuted by the devil.
Delusions of guilt	Delusions of having committed a crime or having sinned greatly – for example, being personally responsible for a recent terrorist attack and so deserving severe punishment.
Nihilistic delusions	Delusions that one no longer exists or that one is about to die or suffer a personal catastrophe. In some cases there may be a belief that other people or objects no longer exist or that the world is coming to an end. Nihilistic delusions are more common in depressive psychosis than in schizophrenia.
Somatic delusions	Delusions of being physically ill or having deformed body parts.
Delusions of jealousy	Delusions that one's spouse or partner is being unfaithful. This may also be referred to as 'Othello syndrome'.
Delusions of love	Delusions of being loved by someone who is inaccessible or with whom one has little contact. It is interesting to note that delusions of jealousy are more common in men whereas delusions of love are more common in women, hinting that delusional themes may have some basis in human evolution.
Delusions of misidentification	Delusions that familiar people have been replaced by identical-looking imposters (Capgras delusion), or that they are disguised as strangers (Fregoli delusion).

Positive symptoms correspond to everyman's notion of 'madness', and people with prominent hallucinations or delusions often evoke fear and contempt. Such negative feelings are reinforced by selective reporting in the media of the rare headline tragedies involving people with (usually untreated) mental disorder. The reality is that the vast majority of schizophrenia sufferers are no more likely to pose a risk to others than the average person. On the other hand, they are far more likely to pose a risk to themselves. For instance, they may neglect their safety and personal care, or leave themselves open to emotional, sexual, or financial exploitation.

Cognitive symptoms involve problems with concentration and memory that can make it difficult to register and recall information, and to formulate and communicate thoughts. Cognitive symptoms are often detectable in the early, prodromal phase of schizophrenia before the onset of positive symptoms, and, though less manifest than positive symptoms, can be just as distressing and disabling.

Whereas positive symptoms can be thought of as an excess or distortion of normal functions, negative symptoms can be thought of as a diminution or loss of normal functions. In some cases, negative symptoms dominate the clinical picture; in others, they are altogether absent. Compared with positive symptoms, negative symptoms tend to be more subtle and less noticeable, but also more persistent, and can perdure right through periods of remission, long after any positive symptoms have burnt out.

Negative symptoms are often misconstrued by the general public, and sometimes also by relatives and carers, as indolence or obstinacy, rather than as the manifestations of a mental disorder. For health professionals, they can be difficult to distinguish from symptoms of depression, or from some of the side-effects of antipsychotic drugs.

The course of schizophrenia can vary considerably from one person to another, but is often marked by a number of distinct phases. In the acute ('initial and short-lasting') phase, positive symptoms come to the fore, while any cognitive and negative symptoms that may already be present sink into the background. The sufferer typically reaches a crisis point at which he comes into contact with mental health services. An antipsychotic drug is started and the acute phase resolves, even though residual positive symptoms may remain.

In some cases, the acute phase is preceded by a so-called prodromal phase lasting for anything from days to years and consisting of subtle and non-specific abnormalities or oddities that may be mistaken for depression or normal teenage behaviour.

The case of Valerie is illustrative of the early stages of schizophrenia:

> *Valerie is a 23-year-old anthropology student who shares a house with three other students on her course. According to her housemates, she has been behaving oddly for the past six months, and since the beginning of term four weeks ago she has not attended a single lecture. One month ago, she found out that her close childhood friend, Chloe, died in a motorbike accident. Since then, she has been secluding herself in her room for hours on end, banging on the furniture, and, it seems, shouting to herself. Her housemates eventually persuaded her to see a doctor.*

> *When Valerie arrived at the doctor's surgery, she was so agitated and distressed that she could not reply to most of his questions. However, he was able to make out that she was hearing three or four male voices coming from outside her head, and that the voices were talking together about her, disparaging her, and blaming her*

*for her family's financial problems. She said that the voices belonged
to SAS paratroopers engaged by her parents to destroy her by
putting certain thoughts, such as the thought of cutting her wrists,
into her head.*

*At the end of the consultation, when the doctor stood up to hold the
door open for her, Valerie screamed, "I've seen your belt! They've
sent you to distract me! I can't... I can't fight them anymore!" and
ran out into the waiting area.*

As the acute phase remits, any cognitive and negative symptoms start
to dominate the picture. This chronic ('long-lasting') phase, if it occurs,
can last for a period of several months or even several years, and may
be punctuated by relapses into a state resembling the acute phase. Such
relapses are often caused by a sudden reduction or discontinuation of
antipsychotic medication, substance misuse, or a stressful life event,
although in many cases there is no identifiable trigger.

Complete recovery from schizophrenia is possible, but most often
the illness runs a protracted course punctuated by episodes of
relapse and remission. Overall, the life expectancy of people with
schizophrenia is reduced by about 8-10 years compared to average,
but this gap is narrowing owing to better standards of physical care.
Perhaps surprisingly, the leading cause of death in schizophrenia
is cardiovascular disease. Other important causes of death include
accidents, drug overdoses, and suicide. The suicide rate is of the
order of 5 per cent, although rates of attempted suicide and
self-harm are considerably higher.

Febrile illnesses such as malaria had been observed to temper
psychotic symptoms, and in the early 20th century 'fever therapy'

became a standard treatment for schizophrenia. Psychiatrists attempted to induce fevers in their patients, sometimes by means of injections of sulphur or oil. Other common but questionable treatments included sleep therapy, gas therapy, electroconvulsive therapy, and prefrontal leucotomy (lobotomy), which involved severing the part of the brain that processes emotions. Sadly, many such 'treatments' aimed more at controlling disturbed behaviour than at curing illness or alleviating suffering. In some countries, such as Germany during the Nazi era, the belief that schizophrenia resulted from a 'hereditary defect' led to atrocious acts of forced sterilization and genocide. The first antipsychotic drug, chlorpromazine, first became available in the 1950s. Although far from perfect, it opened up an era of hope and promise for people with schizophrenia.

Neurotransmitters are chemical messengers released by brain cells to communicate with one another and relay signals. Once released, neurotransmitters bind to specific receptors on target brain cells, causing them to react. According to the so-called dopamine hypothesis of schizophrenia, positive symptoms are produced by an increase in the neurotransmitter dopamine in a part of the brain called the mesolimbic tract (Figure 2.2). Support for the dopamine hypothesis comes, in the main, from two observations: (1) drugs such as amphetamines and cannabis that increase the level of dopamine in the mesolimbic tract can exacerbate the positive symptoms of schizophrenia or even induce a schizophrenia-like psychosis; and (2) antipsychotic drugs that are effective in the treatment of positive symptoms block the effects of increased dopamine in the mesolimbic tract. According to the dopamine hypothesis, the negative symptoms of schizophrenia result from a *decrease* in dopamine in another part of the brain called the mesocortical tract.

The dopamine hypothesis has supplied researchers with a basic model of schizophrenia, but says little about the actual cause of the changes in dopamine levels, and can by no means account for all the subtleties and complexities of the illness or its treatment. More recent research has implicated a number of other neurotransmitters such as glutamate and serotonin, although their precise roles remain unclear. It may be that altered levels of dopamine and other neurotransmitters are interrelated, once again raising the age-old problem of the chicken and the egg.

The dopamine hypothesis submits that antipsychotic drugs are effective in the treatment of positive symptoms because they block

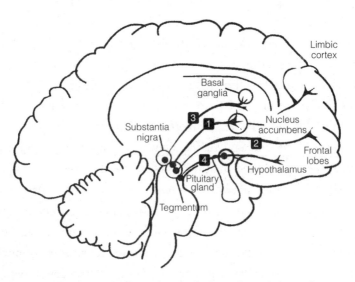

Figure 2.2. The dopamine hypothesis of schizophrenia. According to the dopamine hypothesis, positive symptoms result from an increase of dopamine in the mesolimbic tract (1), while negative symptoms result from a decrease of dopamine in the mesocortical tract (2). The other two dopamine tracts in the brain are the nigrostriatal tract (3), which is affected in Parkinson's disease, and the tuberoinfundibular tract (4).

the action of dopamine in the mesolimbic tract. Unfortunately, they also block the action of dopamine in other brain tracts, commonly leading to a number of unpleasant side-effects such as negative symptoms, disturbances of voluntary muscle function, loss of libido, and erectile dysfunction. Antipsychotic drugs also interfere with neurotransmitters other than dopamine, which can result in further side-effects, first among which sedation and weight gain.

Still, antipsychotics remain the primary treatment for schizophrenia, although psychosocial interventions such as patient and family education, self-help groups, illness self-management, social and vocational skills training, and cognitive-behavioural therapy can all play an important role in reducing symptoms and preventing relapse and re-hospitalization.

Critics of antipsychotic drugs claim that there is nothing specifically 'anti-psychotic' about them, and that they are no more than a form of chemical control, or 'chemical straightjacket'. They highlight that, before being rebranded as 'antipsychotics', the drugs used to be referred to as 'neuroleptics' (a portemanteau coined from the Greek for 'nerve seizure') or 'major tranquillizers'. Physician Henri Laborit (1914-1995) who first trialled chlorpromazine himself described its effect as one of 'artificial hibernation'.

Today, antipsychotic drugs are used not only in the treatment of psychosis, but also, in many cases, in the treatment or management of bipolar disorder, depression, dementia, insomnia, obsessive-compulsive disorder, post-traumatic stress disorder, personality disorder, and autism, among others—suggesting that any effect that they exert is far from targeted.

More specifically, some critics argue that discontinuation-relapse studies overstate the effectiveness of antipsychotic drugs, not least because the drugs sensitize the brain. This means that their discontinuation, especially if sudden, can leave the brain in 'over-drive' and thereby precipitate a relapse. The critics cite, among others, a 20-year longitudinal study led by psychologist Martin Harrow at the University of Illinois which found that longer-term antipsychotic treatment is associated with lower rates of recovery.

Last but not least, critics point out the obvious, which is that antipsychotic drugs often lead to unpleasant and restrictive side-effects, and significantly increase the risk of premature death.

Pioneered in Western Lapland, Finland, the innovative Open Dialogue approach to the management of a mental health crisis, including acute schizophrenia, de-emphasizes antipsychotic drugs. Instead, it focuses on immediate intervention to encourage the person and his family and wider network to come together and talk to one another, in part so that the person may find the words with which to express and lend meaning to his distress. Further studies are planned, but early indications are that the Open Dialogue approach can secure much better treatment outcomes while markedly reducing the use of antipsychotic drugs.

In 1949, neurologist Egas Moniz (1874-1955) received a Nobel Prize for his discovery of 'the therapeutic value of leucotomy in certain psychoses'. Today, prefrontal leucotomy is derided as a barbaric treatment from a much darker age, and it is to be hoped that, one day, so too might antipsychotic drugs.

No single gene can be said to cause schizophrenia. Rather, there are a number of genes that, cumulatively, make a person more or less vulnerable to developing the condition. A person who is highly vulnerable to developing schizophrenia but who lives out a quiet life may be less likely to develop the illness than a person who is only moderately vulnerable but who comes under severe psychological or physical stress.

It is just the same with other conditions such as heart disease or diabetes. Every person inherits a certain complement of genes that makes him more or less vulnerable to developing heart disease. But a person who eats healthily, takes regular exercise, and never smokes is likely to remain healthy almost regardless of his vulnerability. Even if he does develop heart disease, he is likely to do so at an older age and to enjoy a better outcome.

Genes for potentially debilitating illnesses such as schizophrenia typically become less common over time because affected people suffer from a so-called procreative disadvantage, that is, they tend to have fewer children, or fewer healthy children, and so the responsible genes gradually pass out of the population. The fact that this has not happened for schizophrenia suggests that the genes that predispose to the illness are being selected for despite their potentially debilitating effects on a significant proportion of the population, and thus they must be conferring some kind of important adaptive or evolutionary advantage.

It has been suggested that this advantage is no less than our distinctly human abilities for language and creativity. According to psychiatrist Tim Crow of the University of Oxford, our vulnerability to developing schizophrenia arises from the evolution of the human brain to accommodate a language centre in the left hemisphere of the brain. This lateralization of function leads to an anatomical asymmetry in the brain, subtle deviations in which predispose to psychotic symptoms.

In support of this theory, it has been found that psychotic symptoms are associated with a reduction in the usual dominance of the left hemisphere and higher levels of activation in the right hemisphere. Moreover, children with poorly lateralized brains ('hemispheric indeterminism') are at a higher risk of developing schizophrenia, and also of suffering from reading, social, and behavioural problems.

As Prof Crow's theory predicts, schizophrenia is an inherently human illness from which other animals do not seem to suffer. While it is possible to reproduce some of the symptoms of schizophrenia in animals, it has so far proven impossible to reproduce anything like the illness itself.

Communication does not require language, and many animals communicate effectively through more primitive modes of communication. However, language is closely associated with symbolism, and so with emotionalism and creativity. These unique assets not only make us by far the most adaptable of all animals, but also enable us to engage in highly abstract pursuits such as art, music, and religion, and thereby define us as human beings. If our vulnerability to schizophrenia arises from the evolution of language in the human brain, then schizophrenia is, quite literally, the price that we pay for being human. To quote Prof Crow, 'Schizophrenia is not just an illness of humans, it may be THE illness of humanity.'

In the beginning was the Word, and the Word was with God, and the Word was God.

—John 1:1 (KJV)

There are other instances of genes that both predispose to an illness and confer an important adaptive advantage. For example, in sickle cell disease, red blood cells assume a rigid sickle shape that restricts their passage through tiny blood vessels. This leads to a number of serious physical complications and, in the absence of modern medicine, to a radically curtailed life expectancy. At the same time, carrying just one allele of the sickle cell gene ('sickle cell trait') makes it impossible for malarial parasites to reproduce inside red blood cells, and thereby confers immunity to malaria. That the gene for sickle cell disease is commonest in populations from malarial regions suggests that, at least in evolutionary terms, a debilitating illness in the few can be a price worth paying for an important adaptive advantage in the many.

Some highly creative people have suffered from schizophrenia, including Syd Barrett (1946-2006), the early driving force behind the rock band Pink Floyd; John Nash (1928-2015), the father of game theory; and Vaslav Nijinsky (1889-1950), the legendary dancer and choreographer.

In 1912, Nijinsky made his choreographic debut with *Afternoon of a Faun*, set to music by Claude Debussy. On the final scene of erotic masturbation, the sculptor Auguste Rodin remarked that 'nothing could be more striking than the impulse with which, at the climax, he lies face down on the secreted veil, kissing it and hugging it with passionate abandon...' In 1919, Nijinsky's mental health deterio-rated to such an extent that he could no longer dance, and by the time of his death in 1950 he had spent over 30 years in hospital.

John Nash began suffering from schizophrenia during his college years. Despite this, he persevered with his studies, and, in 1994, received the Nobel Prize for economics for 'the pioneering analysis of equilibria in the theory of non-competitive games' (game theory). His life and struggle inspired the biography *A Beautiful Mind*, which was made into a successful Hollywood film.

The cases of Nash and Nijinsky are, however, exceptional, and many people with schizophrenia are intensely disabled by their symptoms. Even highly creative people with schizophrenia tend to be incapacitated during active phases of the illness, while being much more productive before its onset and during later phases of remission.

Many more highly creative people, while not themselves suffering from schizophrenia, have close relatives who do or did. Albert Einstein's son suffered from schizophrenia, as did Bertrand Russell's son and James Joyce's daughter.

Several studies suggest that relatives of schizophrenia sufferers enjoy above average creative intelligence, and one recent family study of 300,000 people with severe mental disorder found that individuals with bipolar disorder and healthy siblings of people with schizophrenia or bipolar disorder are overrepresented in creative professions.

According to one theory, both people with schizophrenia and their non-affected relatives lack lateralization of function in the brain. While this tends to handicap the former, it tends to benefit the latter, who gain in creativity from increased use of the right hemisphere and increased communication between the right and left hemispheres. This increased inter-hemispheric communication also occurs in schizophrenia sufferers, but their cognitive processes tend to be too disorganized for them to make productive use of it.

Some healthy relatives of schizophrenia sufferers may be so close to schizophrenia on the spectrum of normality as to meet the diagnostic criteria for schizotypal personality disorder (see Chapter 1). Many more relatives who do not meet the threshold for schizotypal disorder may nonetheless have mild schizotypal traits, such as divergent or idiosyncratic thinking, which are linked with creativity.

In 2005, Folley and Park at Vanderbilt University conducted a pair of experiments to compare the creative thinking processes of schizophrenia sufferers, 'schizotypes', and normal control subjects. In the first experiment, they asked subjects to make up new functions for household objects. While the schizophrenia sufferers and normal control subjects performed similarly to one another, the schizotypes performed better than either.

In the second experiment, Folley and Park asked the subjects once again to make up new functions for household objects as well as to perform a basic control task while the activity in their prefrontal lobes was monitored by a brain scanning technique called near-infrared optical spectroscopy. While all three groups used both hemispheres for creative tasks, the right hemispheres of schizotypes showed hugely increased activation compared with those of the schizophrenia sufferers and normal control subjects.

For Folley and Park, these results support the idea that increased use of the right hemisphere, and thus increased inter-hemispheric communication, may be related to enhanced creativity in psychosis-prone populations.

In the same year, Nettle and Clegg at the University of Newcastle recruited 425 subjects from specialist creative groups and the general population, and asked them questions designed to measure schizotypal traits, artistic output, and mating success. They found that people who rated highly for 'unusual experiences' and 'impulsive non-conformity' had a higher artistic output and more sexual partners. Those professionally involved in the arts had an average of 5.5 partners, compared to just over 4 for the less creative study participants. It might be that very creative people are seen as more sexually attractive, or that they tend to act more on sexual impulses and opportunities. Whatever the reason or reasons, it could explain how the genes that predispose to schizophrenia are being selected and maintained despite their potentially debilitating effects on a significant proportion of the population.

'Psychosis' is a general term for a mental state involving a loss of contact with reality, as manifested by delusions, hallucinations, or both. This mental state can result from schizophrenia, but also from mood disorders such as depression and bipolar disorder; other mental disorders such as 'brief psychotic disorder'; organic disorders such as temporal lobe epilepsy, brain tumour, stroke, and dementia; drugs such as amphetamines, cocaine, cannabis, and LSD; and stressful or emotionally intense or disturbing experiences.

Brief psychotic disorder looks similar to acute-phase schizophrenia, but is characterized by a rapid onset, vivid delusions or hallucinations, a short course of less than one month (by definition), and a complete recovery. In France, psychiatrists refer to this condition as *bouffée délirante aiguë*, and are apt to describe it as *un coup de tonnerre dans un ciel serein*—'a thunderclap in a clear sky'.

Psychosis can be a non-specific marker of a serious underlying disorder. But it can also represent one end of a continuum of normal human experiences. Hallucinations in particular are very common. In a survey of samples representative of the general population in the UK, Germany, and Italy, as many as 38.7 per cent of respondents reported having experienced hallucinations of one kind or other. In many cases, psychotic phenomena are nothing more than an expression of severe stress or profound emotion, often underlain by a complex, difficult, or deep-seated life problem. In some cases, they may even be a normal or life-enhancing experience, as in, for instance, hearing the comforting voices of ancestors or guardian angels, or seeing visions that are a source of inspiration or revelation.

There can be no doubt that some people have had unusual experiences of different realities at some point in their lives, and been enriched rather than damaged or impaired by them. In a 2006 interview for the Observer, philosopher Robert Pirsig (born 1928), author of *Zen and the Art of Motorcycle Maintenance*, revealed that he refers to his own breakdown both as 'catatonic schizophrenia' and 'hard enlightenment': 'I have never insisted on either, in fact I switch back and forth depending on who I am talking to.'

The idea that psychosis or 'madness' and inspiration and revelation are closely related is an old and recurring one.

For instance, in Plato's *Phaedrus*, which dates back to the 4th century BC, Socrates says:

> *Madness, provided it comes as the gift of heaven, is the channel by which we receive the greatest blessings … the men of old who gave things their names saw no disgrace or reproach in madness; otherwise they would not have connected it with the name of the noblest of arts, the art of discerning the future, and called it the*

> *manic art ... So, according to the evidence provided by our*
> *ancestors, madness is a nobler thing than sober sense ... madness*
> *comes from God, whereas sober sense is merely human.*

In *De Tranquillitate Animi*, Seneca the Younger (4 BC-65 AD) writes that, *nullum magnum ingenium sine mixtuae dementiae fuit* ('there is no great genius without a tincture of madness')—a sentence which he attributes to Aristotle, and which is also echoed in Cicero.

For Shakespeare (1564-1616), 'the lunatic, the lover, and the poet are of imagination all compact.'

And for Dryden (1631-1700), 'great wits are sure to madness near allied, and thin partitions do their bounds divide.'

Despite its age and pedigree, the idea of an intimate relationship between psychosis and inspiration and revelation is, today more than ever, a marginal one. In countries such as the US and UK, people with psychotic symptoms are far more likely to be stigmatized and isolated than tolerated or even celebrated. In contrast, in many traditional societies these same people may be revered as visionaries and mystics, and sought out for their superhuman insights and abilities.

Interestingly, increased use of the right hemisphere is also a feature of healthy people with strong paranormal and religious beliefs. In traditional societies, people with increased use of the right hemisphere, including, of course, people with psychosis, may project an aura of spirituality and mysticism, and, as a result, share in a special, shaman-like status.

The term 'shaman' is generally used to refer to healers, medicine men, seers, sorcerers, and such like, important people whose role within a traditional society may include physical and psychological healing, divining the weather, following totemic animals, communing with the spirits, and placating the gods.

In modern societies, the niche once occupied by the shaman came to be filled first by the priest, and then, ironically, by the psychiatrist.

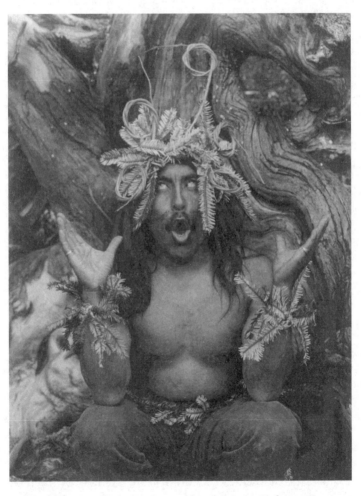

Figure 2.3. Hamatsa shaman possessed by a supernatural power.

Indeed, the term 'psychiatrist' derives from the Greek *psyche* ('soul') and *iatros* ('healer'), and so literally means 'healer of the soul'.

Rather than being stigmatized and isolated, people with schizophrenia and schizotypal traits may be seen as gifted or blessed, and accorded an important social role and attending high social status. That the illness has a better outcome in traditional societies may have much to do with the fact that people living in these tightknit communities see mental disorder more as a part of life than a sign of illness or failure, and enable people with conditions that might otherwise be diagnosed as mental disorder to occupy an honourable place in their very midst.

The current DSM-5 diagnostic criteria for schizophrenia can be summarized as follows:

- First, the person must have at least two characteristic symptoms from a list of five: delusions, hallucinations, disorganized speech, disorganized behaviour, and negative symptoms. One of these two symptoms must be either delusions, hallucinations, or disorganized speech.
- Second, these symptoms must have been present for at least one month, and signs of disturbance for at least six months.
- Third, the symptoms must undermine the person's ability to function in his social or occupational setting.
- Fourth, other psychiatric and medical conditions that can present like schizophrenia—such as drug intoxication, mood disorders, and head injury—must have been excluded.

The majority of medical conditions are defined by their cause ('aetiology') or by the bodily damage that they result in or from ('pathology'), and so are relatively easy to define and recognize. For instance, if someone is suspected of having malaria, a blood sample can be taken and examined under a microscope for malarial parasites of the genus *Plasmodium*; and if someone appears to have suffered a stroke, a brain scan can be taken to look for evidence of obstruction of an artery in the brain. In contrast, mental disorders such as schizophrenia cannot (as yet?) be defined according to their aetiology or pathology, but only according to their manifestations or symptoms. This means that they are more difficult to describe and diagnose, and more open to misunderstanding and misuse.

If a person is suspected of having schizophrenia, there are no laboratory or physical tests that can objectively confirm the diagnosis. Instead, the psychiatrist is left to base his diagnosis on nothing but the person's symptoms, without the support of any tests. If the symptoms tally with the diagnostic criteria for schizophrenia, the psychiatrist is justified in making a diagnosis of schizophrenia.

The problem here is one of circularity: the concept of schizophrenia is defined according to the symptoms of schizophrenia, which in turn are defined according to the concept of schizophrenia. Thus, it is impossible to be sure that 'schizophrenia' maps into any real or distinct disease entity. Given the 'menu of symptoms' approach to diagnosis, it is even possible for two people with no symptoms in common to receive the same label of schizophrenia. Perhaps for this reason, a diagnosis of schizophrenia is a poor predictor of either the severity of the condition or its likely outcome or prognosis.

What's more, psychotic symptoms may form an inadequate basis for diagnosing schizophrenia, since delusions and hallucinations occur in a number of different disorders and states, and therefore represent relatively non-specific indicators of mental disorder. Most of the disability associated with schizophrenia is related to chronic cognitive and negative symptoms, not acute, albeit more florid, positive symptoms. Thus, diagnosing schizophrenia on the basis of psychosis is akin to diagnosing pneumonia on the basis of nothing more than a fever.

Both clinical practice and research into the causes of mental disorders suggest that many of the concepts delineated in classifications of mental disorders, including schizophrenia, depression, and bipolar disorder, do not in fact map onto any real or distinct entities, as Kraepelin led us to believe, but instead lie at different extremes of a single spectrum of mental disorders or states.

Even assuming that the concept of schizophrenia is valid, the symptoms and clinical manifestations that define it are open to interpretation. Recent studies have found that, in reaching a diagnosis of schizophrenia, the rate of agreement between any two independent assessors, that is, the inter-rater reliability, is 65 per cent *at most*. So the concept of schizophrenia is lacking not only in validity, but also in reliability.

That this is so is a consequence of the empirical challenges of investigating the brain, but also, and above all, of the conceptual challenges of understanding the structure and content of human experience. Unfortunately, psychiatric research focuses almost entirely on investigating the brain and hardly at all on rethinking mental disorders or, indeed, rethinking itself. This is, in part, because psychiatry has been reductively classified as a branch of medicine, with many psychiatrists eager to shore up their medical and scientific credentials and unable or reluctant to see beyond the medical model in which they have been schooled.

While a lack of validity and reliability is a problem for all mental disorders, it is a particular problem for schizophrenia, which has a history of being abused for political purposes. In the early 1970s, it became apparent that political and religious dissidents in the Soviet Union were being incarcerated in maximum-security psychiatric hospitals. In 1989, the Soviets authorized a delegation of US psychiatrists to visit certain hospitals and conduct extensive interviews on 27 suspected victims of abuse, of whom 24 had at some time been diagnosed with schizophrenia. This investigation provided unequivocal proof that psychiatry had been abused to incarcerate people whose only transgression had been to oppose the regime. In 14 of the 27 cases, the US team found no evidence of mental disorder of any kind, let alone mental disorder of a nature and degree warranting involuntary detention and treatment. Living conditions in the hospitals were primitive and highly restrictive, with 'patients' unable to keep books or writing materials, and subjected to physical restraints and high-dose injections of antipsychotic and other drugs.

In a paper dating back to 2002, Prof Richard Bonnie writes, 'In some cases, abuse was undoubtedly attributable to intentional misdiagnosis and to knowing complicity by individual psychiatrists in an officially directed effort to repress dissident behaviour. In other cases, the elastic conception of mental disorder used in Soviet psychiatry was probably bent to political purposes, with individual psychiatrists closing their eyes to whatever doubts they may have had about the consequences of their actions.' At the time, the prevailing diagnostic system in the Soviet Union accommodated a very broad concept of schizophrenia, which included mild ('latent' or 'sluggish') and moderate forms characterized by 'personality changes'.

Sadly, such blatant abuse of psychiatry is not confined to the former Soviet Union. China, for one, has established a system of maximum-security psychiatric hospitals (*Ankang*), in part for confining political dissidents and Falun Gong practitioners who represent a 'social danger'. According to a US Department of State report on human rights in China, still in 2014 'there were widespread reports of activists and petitioners being committed to mental health facilities and involuntarily subjected to psychiatric treatment for political reasons.'

The risks of abuse and mistakes are much higher under authoritarian regimes, not least because institutional safeguards such as a strong professional culture among psychiatrists, an independent judiciary, and an open appeals procedure are lacking. But mistakes can take place, and abuse can happen, even under the most liberal of regimes, because, ultimately, a diagnosis of schizophrenia rests on nothing more concrete than subjective opinion.

A delusion is defined as 'a strongly held belief that is not amenable to logic or persuasion and that is out of keeping with its holder's background or culture'. But for a strongly held belief to be a delusion, exactly how strongly must it be held? To whose logic must it not be amenable? And at what precise point is it out of keeping with its holder's background?

In the words of the philosopher and mystic Rajneesh (Osho):

> *There are fictions when the society supports you, there are fictions where nobody supports you. That is the difference between a sane and an insane person; a sane person is one whose fiction is supported by the society. He has manipulated the society to support his fiction. An insane man is one whose fiction is supported by nobody; he is alone so you have to put him in the madhouse.*

In the early 1970s, Prof David Rosenhan (1929-2012) of Stanford University and seven colleagues briefly feigned auditory hallucinations in an attempt to gain admission to various psychiatric hospitals. All eight pseudo-patients were admitted and diagnosed with schizophrenia or, in one case, bipolar disorder. Once admitted, the pseudo-patients acted normally, telling staff that the voices had stopped and that they felt fine. Despite this, staff interpreted much of their behaviour in terms of mental illness. For example, a nurse labelled the note-taking of one pseudo-patient as pathological 'writing behaviour'. The pseudo-patients spent from 7 to 52 days (average 19 days) in hospital, and only secured their release after admitting to mental illness and agreeing to take antipsychotic medication.

In a secondary study, the staff at one hospital was informed that, over the next three months, one or more pseudo-patients would attempt to be admitted into their hospital. Out of 193 new patients, the staff confidently picked out 41 imposters. But Rosenhan had sent no one.

The anti-psychiatry movement took hold in the 1960s and early 1970s, and arose from the difficulties with defining and diagnosing mental disorder. Spearheaded by psychiatrist Thomas Szasz (1920-2012) and others, it claimed that the label of severe mental disorder, especially schizophrenia, was little more than an attempt to medicalize and thereby control socially undesirable behaviour. According to Szasz, 'schizophrenia' does not exist other than as a social construct, a convenient label for the sort of thinking and behaviour that society finds uncomfortable or undermining.

This is rather similar to the opinion of philosopher, historian, and sociologist Michel Foucault (1926-1984), one of the forerunners of the anti-psychiatry movement. One of Foucault's central arguments is that 'madness' is a social construct dating back to the enlightenment, and that its 'treatment' is little more than a disguised form of punishment for deviating from social norms and expectations.

Attractive though it may originally have seemed, the anti-psychiatry claim has been progressively undermined, ultimately, by its reluctance to recognize the distress and suffering of many people with severe mental disorder, as well as the very real risk that they can pose to their safety and prospects.

Of particular note is that Szasz rejected the anti-psychiatry label on the grounds that he did not oppose psychiatric treatment *per se*, but merely held that psychiatric treatment should not be imposed without the consent of the patient.

Today, there can be little doubt that severe mental disorder does, of course, exist, but its nature remains unclear, and an understanding of its place in human affairs—of its meaning—is still sorely lacking, not least because many psychiatrists are reluctant to engage in that debate.

In a different vein from Foucault and Szasz, the psychiatrists RD Laing (1927-1989), Silvano Arieti (1914-1981), and Theodore Lidz (1910-2001) argued that mental disorder is a comprehensible reaction to the impossible demands that families and societies place upon certain sensitive individuals. Laing presented eleven case studies of people with a diagnosis of schizophrenia, and argued that, in each case, the content of their statements and actions was cogent and meaningful in the context of their particular life situation.

Laing never denied the existence of mental disorder, but simply regarded it in a radically different light from his contemporaries. For Laing, the content of a person's psychotic experience was shrouded in an enigmatic language of symbolism that could be interpreted and worked through, rather than overlooked as a meaningless marker of distress or disease. In that much, psychosis can be compared to a waking dream, or, all too often, a waking nightmare.

Why, asked Carl Jung, 'is the mind compelled to expend itself in the elaboration of pathological nonsense?'

> *Our new method of approach gives us a clue to this difficult question. Today we can assert that the pathological ideas dominate the interests of the patient so completely because they are derived from the most important questions that occupied him when he was normal. In other words, what in insanity is now an incomprehensible jumble of symptoms was once a vital field of interest to the normal personality.*

By helping his patient to make sense of his psychotic experience, a psychiatrist may help him not only to feel less alone and alienated, but also to identify and address the source of his distress, and, in so doing, to gain important insights into himself and into life in general. In other words, the psychiatrist may facilitate the conversion of a psychotic episode into a transformative and therapeutic journey akin to that undertaken by the medicine man or shaman.

Chapter 3

Depression, the curse of the strong

And I gave my heart to know wisdom, and to know madness and folly: I perceived that this also is vexation of spirit. For in much wisdom is much grief: and he that increaseth knowledge increaseth sorrow.

—Ecclesiastes 1:17-18 (KJV)

People colloquially use the term 'depression' to refer to normal disappointment or sadness, although in severe cases depression can lead to psychotic symptoms and even death through self-neglect or suicide.

The symptoms of depression can be divided into three groups: core symptoms, psychological symptoms, and physical symptoms (Table 3.1).

Table 3.1: **Symptoms of depression**	
Core symptoms	Low mood Loss of interest or pleasure
Psychological symptoms	Poor concentration Poor self-esteem Inappropriate guilt Recurring thoughts of death or suicide
Physical symptoms	Sleep disturbance Loss of appetite and weight loss Fatigability Agitation or retardation

In contrast to mere disappointment or sadness, the symptoms of depression vary little from day to day and barely respond to changing circumstances. A depressed person who is normally passionate about his work will not brighten up even upon learning that his efforts and achievements have just been recognized with an award that he had long been coveting.

According to DSM-5, for a diagnosis of depression to be made, five or more symptoms from a list similar to the one in Table 3.1 must have been present for a period of two weeks or more. At least one of the symptoms must be either depressed mood or loss of interest or pleasure, and the symptoms must be associated with significant distress or impairment. The diagnostician must also exclude physical states that can masquerade as depression, such as hypothyroidism, anaemia, and drug side-effects.

Severe depression is characterized by intense negative feelings and physical agitation or retardation (slowing down of speech and movements). Retardation is more typical than agitation, although in some cases both can be found in the same person. On occasion, retardation may be so severe that the person is mute and stuporous (motionless and apathetic).

A substantial minority of people with severe depression also suffer from psychotic symptoms (see Chapter 2). Severe depression with psychotic symptoms is often referred to as 'psychotic depression' or 'depressive psychosis'. Psychotic symptoms in depression are usually mood-congruent, that is, in keeping with a depressive outlook. Delusions are commonly along themes of guilt or poverty. Delusions of guilt involve the belief that one has committed a crime or sinned greatly, for instance, by being personally responsible for an earthquake or terrorist attack that has been on the news. Delusions of poverty involve the belief that one is being, or has been, ruined, for instance, by being defrauded by a relative or pursued by a horde of creditors.

Delusions can also take on 'nihilistic' overtones. *Nihil* is Latin for 'nothing', and nihilistic delusions involve the belief that one is about to be reduced to nothing, that is, to die or suffer a personal catastrophe, or even that one is already dead. *Délire de négation* or Cotard's syndrome refers to the combination of nihilistic delusions and somatic delusions (delusions about the body). For instance, a person might believe that his guts are putrefying, or that he has lost all his blood or internal organs. Paranoid delusions, religious delusions, and delusions on other themes are also possible (see Chapter 2, Table 2.2).

In psychotic depression, hallucinations are often of one or several voices, either talking to the person or about the person. The voices are often mocking or attacking, seeking to undermine the person's self-esteem or entrench existing feelings of guilt or hopelessness. Voices that order the person to do certain things are sometimes referred to as 'command hallucinations', and are of particular concern if they are goading the person to harm himself, or, more unusually, other people.

Writer William Styron (1925-2006), the author of *Sophie's Choice*, wrote about his experience of severe depression in *Darkness Visible: A Memoir of Madness*:

> *In depression, this faith in deliverance, in ultimate restoration, is absent. The pain is unrelenting, and what makes the condition intolerable is the foreknowledge that no remedy will come—not in a day, an hour, a month, or a minute. If there is mild relief, one knows that it is only temporary; more pain will follow. It is hopelessness even more than pain that crushes the soul. So the decision-making of everyday life involves not, as in normal affairs, shifting from one annoying situation to another less annoying—or from discomfort to relative comfort, or from boredom to activity— but moving from pain to pain. One does not abandon, even briefly, one's bed of nails, but is attached to it wherever one goes.*

Owing to suicidal ideation, retardation or stupor, food and drink refusal, or psychotic symptoms such as command hallucinations and nihilistic delusions, people with severe depression are often at high risk to themselves. If their level of risk is particularly high, they may be prescribed a course of electroconvulsive therapy (ECT, or 'shock treatment').

It had long been known that convulsions induced by camphor could temper psychotic symptoms. In 1933, psychiatrist Manfred Sakel

(1900-1957) began using insulin injections to induce convulsions, but a period of panic and impending doom prior to convulsing made the treatment very difficult to tolerate. Psychiatrist Ladislas Meduna (1896-1964) replaced the insulin with a drug called metrazol, but similar problems persisted. Then in 1938, neuropsychiatrist Ugo Cerletti (1877-1963) started the practice of applying a small electric shock to the head. This method, which people found more tolerable—or, rather, less intolerable—soon superseded the injections.

In the 1950s, the advent of short-acting anaesthetics and muscle relaxants made it possible for people to be put to sleep for the treatment, and dramatically reduced complications such as muscle tears and bone fractures.

Since the 1950s, several different classes of antidepressant drugs have been introduced, but ECT is still occasionally used as an alternative or supplementary form of treatment, particularly in people with severe depression who are at a high and immediate risk to themselves, or whose condition has not improved after several trials of antidepressant drugs.

During ECT treatment, the person is given a standard anaesthetic and a muscle relaxant. In the UK, the seizure is induced with a constant current, brief-pulse stimulus at a voltage that is just above the person's seizure threshold. The seizure typically lasts for about 30 seconds, and in many cases is so unremarkable that it can only be witnessed on the monitor of an electroencephalogram (EEG), which is a device for recording the electrical activity of the brain.

In the UK, most people who are prescribed ECT are prescribed a course of between six and twelve treatments, usually delivered over the course of three to six weeks.

Common side-effects of ECT include nausea, muscle aches, headache, confusion, and memory loss for events that occurred around the time of the treatment. Mortality from ECT is largely imputable to the anaesthetic, and is similar to that for any minor surgical procedure.

Opinion is divided as to the effectiveness and value of ECT. Several studies lend weight to the frequent anecdotal reports that ECT can be considerably more effective than antidepressant treatment.

However, opponents claim that the evidence in support of ECT is weak, and that any benefits are short-lived and outweighed by the risks, including the risk of long-term memory impairment. They also highlight that, despite decades of research, proponents of ECT cannot point, or point with certainty, to a mechanism of action for its antidepressant effect.

In addition to these criticisms, ECT suffers from a poor public image. For decades, the media has, more often than not, portrayed it as coercive, punitive, and inhumane. A case in point is the classic film *One Flew Over the Cuckoo's Nest*. Adapted from Ken Kasey's popular 1962 novel by the same name, it stars Jack Nicholson as the spirited RP McMurphy ('Mac') and Louise Fletcher as the chilly but softly spoken Nurse Ratched. When Mac arrives at the Oregon state mental hospital, he challenges the stultifying routine and bureaucratic authoritarianism personified by Nurse Ratched, and pays the price by being drugged, electroshocked, and, ultimately, lobotomized. While the film is highly successful as a metaphor of total institutions—that is, institutions that repress individuality to create a compliant society—its portrayal of psychiatric care is both misleading and outdated.

The first antidepressant drug, iproniazid, appeared in the 1950s, some 20 years after ECT. The compound was initially trialled in people with tuberculosis, who were subsequently noted to be 'inappropriately happy'. Iproniazid and other, later drugs in the class of the monoamine oxidase inhibitors (MAOIs) are said to exert their antidepressant effect by preventing the enzymatic breakdown of monoamine neurotransmitters.

Back in the 1950s, MAOIs revolutionized the treatment of depression. However, the drugs also prevent the breakdown of the amino acid tyramine in the gastrointestinal tract, which, through the accumulation of tyramine, can lead to a potentially fatal hypertensive reaction. As a result, people on MAOIs must steer clear from a long list of tyramine-containing foods and beverages, including such staples as beer, cheese, and sausage. For this and other reasons, MAOIs are seldom used today.

Imipramine, the first tricyclic antidepressant, appeared soon after iproniazid. Tricyclics are said to exert their antidepressant effect by preventing the re-uptake of the monoamine neurotransmitters noradrenaline (norepinephrine) and serotonin by brain cells. Unlike with MAOIs, people on tricyclics can eat and drink freely. However, they often suffer from a range of troublesome and potentially dangerous side-effects. Tricyclics are still occasionally prescribed, but, owing to their side-effect profile and high toxicity in overdose, are contraindicated in the elderly, the physically ill, and those at risk of self-harm.

It took another thirty or so years for the next class of antidepressants to make its entry. Fluoxetine, the first selective serotonin reuptake inhibitor (SSRI), only gained regulatory approval in 1987.

SSRIs are said to exert their antidepressant effect by preventing the reuptake of serotonin by brain cells. Compared to tricyclics, they have milder side-effects and are less toxic in overdose. Today, SSRIs such as fluoxetine, fluvoxamine, paroxetine, sertraline, and citalopram are the drugs of choice for most cases of moderate to severe depression. Like antipsychotics, SSRIs have become something of a panacea, and are also used in the treatment of a broad range of other mental disorders, particularly anxiety disorders, obsessive-compulsive disorder, and bulimia nervosa, and even in some physical disorders such as premature ejaculation in young men and hot flushes in menopausal women. In the UK, the SSRI fluoxetine is so commonly prescribed that trace quantities have been detected in the drinking water.

Since 1987, further classes of antidepressants have been developed, such as the noradrenaline reuptake inhibitors (NARIs) and the serotonin and noradrenaline reuptake inhibitors (SNRIs). These more recent types of antidepressant are often used as second-line treatments if treatment with an SSRI has failed, but their precise role in the management of depression remains to be established.

People starting on an SSRI are usually told to persist in taking their tablets because improvement in mood may be delayed for 10-20 days (in which time mood may have improved of its own accord), and because potential side-effects are likely to be only mild and short-lived. These side-effects include nausea, diarrhoea, dizziness, agitation, and sexual dysfunction. Suddenly stopping an SSRI can provoke a discontinuation syndrome consisting of mild and non-specific symptoms. This has led to the suggestion that SSRIs are 'addictive', but this is not strictly accurate in the sense that people do not experience a buzz from SSRIs, and do not crave them as they might a drug of abuse such as cocaine or heroin. There are also some reports that SSRIs cause, or are associated with, increased suicidal thoughts and behaviours in children and young people, but the studies looking into this remain equivocal and the jury is still out.

Doctors often assure people starting on an SSRI that they have about a 50-70 per cent chance of responding to their medication. However, in 2008, a study published in the *New England Journal of Medicine* suggested that the effectiveness of SSRIs is greatly exaggerated owing to a bias in the reporting of research studies. Out of 74 studies registered with the US Food and Drug Administration (FDA), 37 out of 38 studies with positive results were published in academic journals, compared to only 14 out of 36 studies with negative results. Moreover, out of the 14 studies with negative results that were published, 11 were published in such a way as to convey a positive outcome. Thus, while 94 per cent (37+11/37+14) of published studies conveyed a positive outcome, only 51 per cent (38/38+36) of all studies, published and unpublished, actually demonstrated one.

Another piece of research published in the *Public Library of Science*, also in 2008, combined 35 studies submitted to the FDA before the licensing of four antidepressants including the SSRIs fluoxetine and paroxetine. The researchers found that, while the antidepressants performed better than a placebo, the effect size was very small for all but the very severe cases of depression. Moreover, the researchers attributed this increased effect size in very severe cases of depression not to an actual increase in the effect of the antidepressants, but to a decrease in their placebo effect.

If, as these studies suggest, the effectiveness of SSRIs has been greatly exaggerated, their cost-benefit urgently needs to be re-evaluated.

In any case, there can be little doubt that at least some of the benefit of antidepressants stems from their placebo effect. The term 'placebo effect' derives from the Latin *placare* ('to please'), and refers to the tendency for a remedy to 'work' simply because it is expected to.

One leading theory explains the placebo effect in terms of classical, or Pavlovian, conditioning.

In an unconditioned reflex, an unconditioned stimulus (UCS, for example, food) triggers an unconditioned response (UCR, for example, salivation).

$$UCS \quad = \quad UCR$$
$$Food \quad = \quad Salivation$$

In a conditioned reflex, a neutral stimulus (NS, for example, the ringing of a bell) is repeatedly paired with the UCS, as a result of which the neutral stimulus, now a conditioned stimulus (CS), can also trigger the UCR, now a conditioned response (CR).

$$UCS \quad + \quad NS \qquad = \quad UCR$$
$$Food \quad + \quad Bell \qquad = \quad Salivation$$
$$\qquad\qquad NS\,(CS) \quad = \quad UCR\,(CR)$$
$$\qquad\qquad Bell \qquad = \quad Salivation$$

The above paradigm echoes the classical experiment first carried out by physiologist Ivan Pavlov (1849-1936) on dogs. Psychologist John B. Watson (1878-1958) elaborated on Pavlov's findings by demonstrating, through his famous 'little Albert experiment', that conditioning can also extend to emotions.

Each time a loud bang was produced, the nine-month old Albert became frightened and cried.

UCS	=	UCR
Loud bang	=	Fear

Later, an experimental rat was introduced; but each time Albert tried to pet the rat, the loud bang was reproduced. After one week and just seven pairings, the rat was presented to Albert on its own, without the loud bang. But by then Albert had become frightened of the rat, and recoiled from it.

UCS	+	NS	=	UCR
Loud bang	+	Rat	=	Fear
		NS (CS)	=	UCR (CR)
		Rat	=	Fear

Returning to the placebo effect, the idea is that people who associate taking a remedy with improvement may come to expect improvement if they take a remedy, even if the 'remedy' in question is no more than an inert substance, or a substance that has no therapeutic effect but only 'side-effects' that can be interpreted as indicative of a therapeutic effect. It may be that the expectation alone suffices to mimic the effect of the remedy, and brain imaging studies indicate that, in some cases, remedies and their placebos can activate the very same mechanisms in the nervous system.

Remedies that are perceived to be more potent tend to have a stronger placebo effect. Perceptions of potency are influenced by a multitude of factors, including the remedy's size, shape, colour, route of administration, and general availability. Perceptions of potency are also influenced by the person recommending or administering the remedy, such that a remedy recommended by a doctor tends to have a stronger placebo effect than one recommended by a nurse, pharmacist, or layman. This means that a brightly coloured injection administered by a silver-haired professor of medicine can be expected to have a much stronger placebo effect, and therefore a much stronger overall effect, than the drab over-the-counter tablet recommended by the neighbour's teenager. This highlights the importance of the psychological, social, and cultural context in which a treatment is administered, and, more particularly, the significance of the therapeutic act or ritual.

Classical conditioning not only helps to explain the placebo effect, but also underlies psychological treatments such as systemic desensitization therapy and aversion therapy. Systemic desensitization therapy, also known as graduated exposure therapy, is frequently used in the treatment of phobias, and involves introducing the feared object by degrees. For instance, a person with arachnophobia is asked, first, to think about spiders, then to look at pictures of spiders, then to look at real spiders from a safe distance, and so on, while using relaxation exercises at each stage to help control and relieve anxiety.

Aversion therapy is used to discourage problematic behaviours, and involves pairing the unwanted behaviour with an aversive stimulus such as an electric shock or the unpleasant flushing reaction produced by the drug disulfiram (Antabuse) when it is combined with alcohol.

In the 1950s and 1960s, some therapists employed aversion therapy of the kind featured in *A Clockwork Orange* to 'cure' male homosexuality. This typically involved showing 'patients' pictures of naked men while giving them electric shocks or drugs to make them vomit, and, once they could no longer bear it, showing them pictures of naked women or sending them out on a 'date' with a young nurse. Needless to say, these cruel and degrading methods proved entirely ineffective.

First published in 1968, DSM-II listed homosexuality as a mental disorder. In 1973, the American Psychiatric Association (APA) asked all members attending its convention to vote on whether they believed homosexuality to be a mental disorder. 5,854 psychiatrists voted to remove homosexuality from the DSM, and 3,810 voted to retain it. The APA then compromised, removing homosexuality from the DSM but replacing it, in effect, with 'sexual orientation disturbance' for people 'in conflict with' their sexual orientation. Not until 1987 did homosexuality completely fall out of the DSM.

Meanwhile, the World Health Organization (WHO) only removed homosexuality from the ICD with the publication of ICD-10 in 1992, although ICD-10 still carries the construct of 'ego-dystonic sexual orientation'.

The evolution of the status of homosexuality in the classifications of mental disorders highlights that concepts of mental disorder can be social constructs that change as society changes. Today, the standard of psychotherapy in the US and Europe is gay affirmative psychotherapy, which encourages gay people to accept their sexual orientation.

Antidepressants are the most readily available form of treatment for depression, but, very often, psychological treatments can offer a safer and more effective alternative. Many people prefer psychological treatments to antidepressants on the grounds that psychological treatments address underlying problems, whereas antidepressants merely mask superficial symptoms. Their attitude reveals that, despite the predominance of the biological model, they do not think of depression as a biological disorder of the brain, but as a marker of unidentified or unresolved life problems.

At its most basic, psychological treatment involves little more than explanation and reassurance. Such 'supportive therapy' is often sorely lacking, but ought to be offered to all people diagnosed with depression. In people diagnosed with milder forms of depression, supportive therapy is often the only intervention that is either necessary or appropriate.

Counselling is similar to supportive therapy in that it involves explanation, reassurance, and encouragement. However, counselling also aims at identifying and resolving life problems, and so is more problem-focused and goal-oriented than supportive therapy.

In contrast to supportive therapy and counselling, exploratory psychotherapy endeavours to examine the person's thoughts and feelings. Two important, yet very different, forms of exploratory psychotherapy are psychodynamic psychotherapy and cognitive-behavioural therapy (CBT).

Psychodynamic psychotherapy is founded on psychoanalytic theory. It is similar to psychoanalysis, but less intensive and more limited in duration. In contrast to CBT, which is based on learning and cognitive theories, psychodynamic psychotherapy can, and usually does, delve into past and childhood experiences, and is particularly invaluable if the origin of the depression appears to be deep-seated.

According to one influential psychodynamic theory of depression, depression can result in later life if an infant forms an insecure attachment with other persons, usually his mother but often also his father and other significant adults.

Inspired by the seminal work of psychiatrist John Bowlby (1907-1990) on attachment theory, psychologist Mary Ainsworth (1913-1999) devised an experiment called the 'Strange Situation' to observe patterns of attachment in human infants. In the Strange Situation, an infant is observed exploring toys for twenty minutes while his mother and a stranger enter and leave the room at different times. Depending on the infant's behaviour upon being reunited with his mother, he is classified into one of three categories: secure attachment, anxious-ambivalent insecure attachment, and anxious-avoidant insecure attachment.

In secure attachment, the infant explores freely and engages with the stranger while his mother is present. When his mother leaves, he is subdued but not distressed; and when she returns, he greets her positively. A pattern of secure attachment is thought to arise if the mother is generally available and responsive to the infant and able to meet his needs adequately.

In anxious-ambivalent insecure attachment, the infant is anxious of exploration and ambivalent towards the stranger, even in the presence of his mother. When his mother leaves, he is distressed; but when she returns he is ambivalent towards her. A pattern of anxious-ambivalent insecure attachment is thought to arise if the mother generally provides the infant with attention, but only inconsistently and according to her own needs.

Finally, in anxious-avoidant insecure attachment, the infant explores the toys but seems unconcerned by the presence or absence of either the stranger or his mother, although he does not avoid the stranger as strongly as he does his mother. A pattern of anxious-avoidant insecure attachment is thought to arise if the mother generally disengages from the infant, who comes to believe that he cannot exert any influence over his caregiver.

An infant's pattern of attachment is important because it can lead to an internal model of the self as unlovable and inadequate, and of others as unresponsive and punitive. It can also help to predict a person's response to loss or adversity, as well as his pattern of relating to peers, engaging in romantic relationships, and parenting children.

Through the parenting of children, an insecure attachment can be passed on from parent to child, and in this manner one generation's loss can be inherited by the next. That which a child did not receive, he cannot later give; or, as the Talmud puts it:

> *The parent who teaches his son, it is as if he had taught his son, his son's son, and so on to the end of generations.*

—Talmud Kiddushin, 36

In contrast to psychodynamic psychotherapy, CBT focuses exclusively on the here and now. Developed by psychiatrist Aaron Beck (born 1921) in the 1960s, CBT has become a mainstream treatment for non-severe depression and a number of other mental disorders. In the short-term, it is at least as effective as antidepressants, and in the long-term may be more effective than antidepressants at preventing relapses.

CBT is most often carried out on a one-to-one basis, but can also be offered in small groups. It involves a defined number of sessions, typically between ten and twenty, but principally takes place outside of sessions through 'homework'. The person and a trained therapist (who may be a doctor, psychologist, nurse, or counsellor) develop a shared perspective of the person's current problems, and try to understand them in terms of his thoughts (cognitions), emotions, and behaviours, and of how these are likely to relate to one another. This leads to the identification of realistic, time-limited goals, and of cognitive and behavioural strategies for achieving them.

In CBT for depression, cognitive strategies principally aim at modifying automatic and self-perpetuating negative thoughts. These cognitive biases or thinking errors are considered as hypotheses, which, through gentle questioning and guided discovery, can be examined, tested, and modified.

According to Beck, thinking errors are rooted in negative schemas acquired in childhood and adolescence, for example, through the loss of a parent, criticism from parents and teachers, or rejection and bullying by peers. In later life, these negative schemas can be reactivated by any event or circumstance that resembles or recalls the initial trauma.

Three examples of thinking errors in depression are selective abstraction, dichotomous thinking, and catastrophic thinking. Selective abstraction is focusing on a single negative state or event to the exclusion of other, more positive ones. For example, a person may be preoccupied that he is not currently in a relationship, but overlook that he has a supportive family and numerous close friends. Dichotomous thinking is 'all-or-nothing' thinking. A common example of dichotomous thinking in hospital in-patients with depression is, 'if she doesn't come to see me today, this means she doesn't love me.' Another, more subtle, example is, 'if I am not out of hospital by my daughter's birthday, she'll think that I don't love her.' Catastrophic thinking is imagining the worse possible outcome for any problem or situation, for example:

The pain in my knee is getting worse. When I'm reduced to a wheelchair, I won't be able to go to work and pay the mortgage. So I'll end up losing my house and dying in the street.

CBT for depression aims mostly at modifying automatic and self-perpetuating negative thoughts, but it can also involve behavioural tasks and exercises that aim at shaping and reinforcing positive behaviour. These behavioural strategies are based on the principles of both classical conditioning, discussed above, and operant conditioning.

After observing the behaviour of cats attempting to escape from puzzle boxes, psychologist EL Thorndike (1874-1949) formulated the 'law of effect' according to which behaviours that produce positive consequences are 'stamped in' so as to occur with increasing frequency. Psychologist BF Skinner (1904-1990) refined Thorndike's ideas by introducing the concepts of reinforcement and punishment, which are summarized in Table 3.2.

Table 3.2: Four types of operant conditioning			
Type	**Consequence**	**Example**	**Outcome**
Positive reinforcement	Something good is added	Rewarding good behaviour with a prize	Behaviour is stamped in
Negative reinforcement	Something bad is subtracted	Using relaxation techniques to reduce or eliminate anxiety	Behaviour is stamped in
Positive punishment	Something bad is added	Punishing bad behaviour with a slap on the hand	Behaviour is stamped out
Negative punishment	Something good is subtracted	Punishing bad behaviour by locking away the games console	Behaviour is stamped out

According to behavioural psychology, or behaviourism, all behaviours are acquired through conditioning, which occurs exclusively through interaction with the environment. One important implication is that behaviour can be studied empirically, without any need to take account of internal mental states which, by their nature, can be neither observed nor quantified.

In 1930, John B. Watson went so far as to write:

> *Give me a dozen healthy infants, well-formed, and my own specified world to bring them up in and I'll guarantee to take any one at random and train him to become any type of specialist I might select—doctor, lawyer, artist, merchant-chief and, yes, even beggar-man and thief, regardless of his talents, penchants, tendencies, abilities, vocations, and race of his ancestors.*

Although behaviourists did emphasize the role of the environment, their position was not as extreme as this quotation suggests, and in the same statement Watson went on to write, 'I am going beyond my facts and I admit it, but so have the advocates of the contrary and they have been doing so for many thousands of years.'

Being all 'out there', behaviourism is easy to study and put into practise, and is often successful in replacing maladaptive behaviours with more helpful or positive ones. Nonetheless, behaviourism is often criticized for ignoring internal states such as thoughts and feelings, and for neglecting other types of learning such as insight learning, an advanced form of learning which builds upon knowledge and reason to solve a problem or gain a new understanding without the trial and error involved in other types of learning.

In 1967, psychologist Martin Seligman (born 1942) serendipitously found that the conditioning of dogs could lead to outcomes opposite to those predicted by behaviourism. Seligman observed that dogs that had learnt that they could not escape from electric shocks did not try to do so, even when the situation permitted it. In other words, dogs that had learnt that they could not exert control over their environment permanently lost the will or capacity to do so. Extended to human behaviour, this 'learnt helplessness' provided an influential cognitive-behavioural model of depression.

However, Seligman noticed that not *all* the dogs exhibited learnt helplessness, with about one-third successfully escaping from the electric shocks despite their negative past experiences. In humans, Seligman found that learnt helplessness is associated with a 'negative explanatory style'. For example, if my friend Bill got angry about something that I did, I could explain his anger either by saying something like, 'Bill's in a bad mood today, but I'm sure he'll be all right next time I see him' (positive explanatory style), or by saying something like, 'Oh dear, I should never have done that. I'm cold and inconsiderate, and Bill's never going to talk to me again' (negative explanatory style).

According to Seligman, a person's explanatory style can be changed. Learnt helplessness can be replaced with 'learnt optimism' through cognitive strategies similar to those used in CBT for depression, such as identifying negative interpretations of events, evaluating their accuracy, and generating more positive or constructive interpretations.

Learnt helplessness can begin very early in life if an infant is unable to influence the response of his carers through such behaviours as smiling and crying. Later on in life, children often model their behaviour on that of their carers. Thus, a negative explanatory style can be passed on from parent to child, and, in this manner also, one generation's loss can be 'inherited' by the next.

For Seligman, parents can promote learnt optimism in their children by providing them with role models of learnt optimism, allowing them greater control over their environment, and encouraging them to solve problems and acquire a sense of mastery.

CBT for depression has garnered a great deal of institutional support on the basis that it is cheap and effective. However, critics question the robustness of the research into CBT for depression, and claim that it is in fact no more effective than other psychological treatments.

Curiously, one study published in 2015 found that the effectiveness of CBT for depression has been declining ever since the seminal

CBT trials of the 1970s, with the steepest decline in the period from 1995. One explanation might be that, as CBT for depression has become more and more common, the quality of training, or the quality of trained therapists, has declined.

More fundamentally, by leaning so heavily on patterns of cognition, CBT may be mistaking the symptoms of depression for its causes, while implying that depression has little or nothing to do with life circumstances. Moreover, in assuming that people are entirely determined by involuntary or unreflective cognitive processes, CBT denies the possibility of free will or agency. This confused and reductive approach may frustrate and even alienate the person, and contribute to the high drop-out rates observed in CBT for depression.

Some of these concerns are addressed by mindfulness-based cognitive therapy (MBCT), which combines traditional CBT methods with 'newer' psychological strategies such as mindfulness and mindfulness meditation. In essence, mindfulness, which derives from Buddhist spiritual practice, aims at increasing our awareness and acceptance of incoming thoughts and feelings, and so the flexibility or fluidity of our responses, which become less like unconscious reactions and more like conscious reflections. Mindfulness can be harnessed for the treatment of recurrent depression, stress, anxiety, and addiction, among others; but it can also be used to broadly improve our quality of life by decentering us and shifting our focus from doing to being.

Seligman's studies of learnt helplessness demonstrate that thoughts and behaviours associated with depression do not merely exist in a vacuum, but are deeply embedded in past experience. This rootedness is explicitly recognized by psychodynamic psychotherapy, and Beck himself postulated that cognitive biases arise from negative schemas acquired in childhood and adolescence.

Even so, to say that depression is rooted in past experience does not go nearly far enough, for depression is not merely rooted in past experience. It is also rooted in the nature of human experience.

In *Man's Search for Meaning*, psychiatrist and neurologist Victor Frankl (1905-1997) wrote about his ordeal as a concentration camp inmate during the Second World War. Interestingly, he found that those who survived longest in concentration camps were not those who were physically strong, but those who retained a sense of control over their environment.

He observed:

> *We who lived in concentration camps can remember the men who walked through the huts comforting others, giving away their last piece of bread. They may have been few in number, but they offer sufficient proof that everything can be taken from a man but one thing: the last of human freedoms—to choose one's own attitude in any given set of circumstances—to choose one's own way.*

Frankl's message is ultimately one of hope: even in the most absurd, painful, and dispiriting of circumstances, life can be given a meaning, and so too can suffering. Life in the concentration camp taught Frankl that our main drive or motivation in life is neither pleasure, as Freud had believed, nor power, as Adler had believed, but *meaning*.

After his release, Frankl founded the school of logotherapy (from the Greek *logos*, meaning 'reason' or 'principle'), which is sometimes referred to as the 'Third Viennese School of Psychotherapy' for coming after those of Freud and Adler. The aim of logotherapy is to carry out an existential analysis of the person, and, in so doing, to help him uncover or discover meaning for his life.

According to Frankl, meaning can be found through:

- Experiencing reality by interacting authentically with the environment and with others,
- Giving something back to the world through creativity and self-expression, and
- Changing our attitude when faced with a situation or circumstance that we cannot change.

Frankl is credited with coining the term 'Sunday neurosis' to refer to the dejection that many people feel at the end of the working week when at last they have the time to realize just how empty and meaningless their life has become. This existential vacuum may open the door on all sorts of excesses and compensations such as neurotic anxiety, avoidance, binge eating, drinking, overworking, and overspending. In the short-term, these excesses and compensations carpet over the existential vacuum, but in the longer term they prevent action from being taken and meaning from being found.

For Frankl, depression results when the gap between what a person is and what he ought to be, or once wished to be, becomes so large that it can no longer be carpeted over. The person's goals seem far out of reach and he can no longer envisage a future. As in Psalm 41, *abyssus abyssum invocat*—'hell brings forth hell', or, in an alternative translation, 'the deep calls unto the deep.'

In recent decades, depression has become increasingly common in industrialized countries, and is often referred to by doctors as 'the common cold of psychiatry'. Figures for the lifetime risk of developing depression vary according to the criteria used to define the condition. Using DSM-5's criteria for 'Major Depressive Disorder', which are similar to ICD-10's criteria for moderate depression, the lifetime prevalence of depression is about 15 per cent, and the point prevalence about 5 per cent. This means that the average person has a 15 per cent chance of having suffered from depression at some time, and a 5 per chance of suffering from it at this point in time.

These figures mask an uneven gender distribution, with women twice more likely to be diagnosed with depression than men. The reasons for this asymmetry are unclear, and thought to be in parts biological, psychological, and sociocultural.

Possible biological explanations: compared to men, women are subjected to fluctuating hormone levels, particularly around the times of childbirth and the menopause. Beyond this, they might also have a stronger genetic predisposition to developing depression.

Possible psychological explanations: women are more ruminative than men, that is, they tend to think through things more. Men, in contrast, are likelier to respond to life problems with stoicism, anger, or substance misuse. Women also tend to be more invested in relationships, and so more affected and afflicted by relationship issues.

Possible sociocultural explanations: women come under greater stress than men. In addition to going to work just like men, they are often expected to bear most of the burden of maintaining the family home, bringing up the children, and caring for older relatives—and, after all that, they still have to put up with the sexism! Women live longer than men, and extreme old age is often associated with bereavement, loneliness, poor health, and precarity. Finally, women are more likely to seek out a diagnosis of depression than men. They are more likely to consult a doctor and more likely to discuss their feelings with the doctor. Conversely, doctors, whether themselves men or women, may be more inclined to diagnose depression in a woman.

There are also important geographical variations in the prevalence of depression, and these can in large part be accounted for by sociocultural rather than biological factors. In traditional societies, emotional distress is more likely to be interpreted as an indicator of the need to address important life problems rather than as a mental disorder requiring professional treatment, and so a diagnosis of depression is correspondingly less common. Some linguistic communities do not even have a word for 'depression', and many people from traditional societies with what may be construed as depression present instead with physical complaints such as fatigue, headache, or chest pain.

Punjabi women who have recently immigrated to the UK and given birth find it baffling that a health visitor should pop round to ask them if they are depressed, not least because it had never crossed their minds that giving birth could be anything but a joyful event.

Being much more exposed to the concept of depression, people in modern societies such as the UK and US are likelier to interpret their distress in terms of depression and to seek out a diagnosis of the illness. At the same time, groups with vested interests such as pharmaceutical companies and so-called mental health experts actively promote the notion of saccharine happiness as a natural, default state, and of human distress as a mental disorder.

The concept of depression as a mental disorder may be useful for the more severe and intractable cases treated by hospital psychiatrists, but not for the majority of cases, which, for the most part, are mild and short-lived and easily interpreted in terms of life circumstances, human nature, or the human condition.

Another non-mutually exclusive explanation for the important geographical variations in the prevalence of depression may lie in the nature of modern societies, which have become increasingly individualistic and divorced from traditional values. For many people living in our society, life can seem both suffocating and far removed, lonely even and especially among the multitudes, and not only meaningless but absurd. By encoding their distress in terms of a mental disorder, our society is subtly implying that the problem lies not with itself but with them, fragile and failing individuals that they are.

Of course, many people prefer to buy into this reductive explanation than to confront their existential angst. But thinking of their unhappiness in terms of an illness or chemical imbalance can prevent them from identifying and addressing the important psychological or life problems that are at the root of their distress.

All this is not to say that the concept of depression as a mental disorder is bogus, but merely that the diagnosis of depression has been over-extended to include much more than just depression the mental disorder. If, like the majority of medical conditions, depression could be defined and diagnosed according to its aetiology or pathology, such a state of affairs could never have arisen. Unfortunately, depression, like schizophrenia and other mental disorders, cannot be defined according to its aetiology or pathology, but only according to its clinical manifestations or symptoms. This means that a doctor cannot base a diagnosis of depression on any objective criterion such as a blood test or brain scan, but only on his subjective interpretation of the nature and severity of the patient's symptoms. If some of these symptoms appear to tally with the diagnostic criteria for depression, then the physician is able to justify a diagnosis of depression.

As with schizophrenia, the problem is one of circularity: the concept of depression is defined according to the symptoms of depression, which in turn are defined according to the concept of depression. Thus, one cannot be sure that the concept of depression has any biological validity, particularly since a diagnosis of depression can apply to anything from mild depression to depressive psychosis and depressive stupor, and overlap with several other categories of mental disorder, including dysthymia, adjustment disorders, and anxiety disorders.

As it stands, the diagnostic criteria for depression are so loose that two people with absolutely no symptoms in common can both end up with the same unitary diagnosis of depression. For this reason especially, the concept of depression as a mental disorder has been charged with being little more than a socially constructed dustbin for all manner of human suffering.

Let us grant, as the orthodoxy has it, that every person inherits a certain complement of genes that makes him more or less vulnerable to entering a state that could be diagnosed as depression (and let us also refer to this state as 'the depressive position' to include the entire continuum of depressed mood, including but not limited to clinical depression). A person enters the depressive position if the amount of stress that he comes under is greater than the amount of stress that he can tolerate given the complement of genes that he has inherited. Genes for potentially debilitating disorders gradually pass out of a population over time because affected people have, on average, fewer children or fewer healthy children than non-affected people. But the fact that this has not happened for depression suggests that the genes responsible are being maintained despite their potentially debilitating effects on a significant proportion of the population, and thus that they are conferring an important adaptive advantage.

What important adaptive advantage could the depressive position be conferring? Just as physical pain has evolved to signal injury and prevent further injury, so the depressive position could have evolved to remove us from distressing, damaging, or futile situations. The time and space and solitude that the depressive position affords prevent us from making rash decisions, enable us to reconnect with the bigger picture, and encourage us to reassess our social relationships, think about those who matter to us most, and relate to them more meaningfully and compassionately. In other words, the depressive position evolved as a signal that something is seriously wrong and needs working through and changing, or, at the very least, processing and understanding.

Sometimes we can become so immersed in the humdrum of our everyday existence that we no longer have the time to think and feel about ourselves, and so lose sight of our bigger picture. The adoption of the depressive position can force us to cast off the polyannish optimism and rose-tinted spectacles that shield us from reality, stand back at a distance, re-evaluate and prioritize our needs, and formulate a modest but realistic plan for fulfilling them.

At an even deeper level, the adoption of the depressive position can encourage us to develop a more refined perspective and more profound understanding of our self, our life, and life in general. From an existential standpoint, the adoption of the depressive position obliges us to become aware of our mortality and freedom, and challenges us to exercise the latter within the framework of the former. By meeting this difficult challenge, we are able to break out of the mould that has been imposed upon us, discover who we truly are, and, in so doing, begin to give deep meaning to our lives.

Many of the most creative and insightful people in our society suffered from depression or a state that could have met the DSM-V criteria for Major Depressive Disorder. They included the politicians Winston Churchill and Abraham Lincoln; the poets Charles Baudelaire, Elizabeth Bishop, Hart Crane, Emily Dickinson, Sylvia Plath, and Rainer Maria Rilke; the thinkers Michel Foucault, William James, John Stuart Mill, Isaac Newton, Friedrich Nietzsche, and Arthur Schopenhauer; and the writers Agatha Christie, Charles Dickens, William Faulkner, Graham Greene, Leo Tolstoy, Evelyn Waugh, and Tennessee Williams—among many, many others. To quote Marcel Proust, who himself suffered from depression, 'Happiness is good for the body, but it is grief which develops the strengths of the mind.'

People in the depressive position are often stigmatized as 'failures' or 'losers'. Of course, nothing could be further from the truth.

If these people are in the depressive position, it is most probably because they have tried too hard or taken on too much, so hard and so much that they have made themselves 'ill with depression'. That is to say, if these people are in the depressive position, it is because their world was simply not good enough for them. They wanted more, they wanted better, and they wanted different, not just for themselves, but for all those around them. So if they are failures or losers, this is only because they set the bar far too high. They could have swept everything under the carpet and pretended, as many of us do, that all is for the best in the best of possible worlds. But unlike many people, they had the honesty and the strength to admit that something was amiss, that something was not quite right. So rather than being failures or losers, they are all the opposite: they are ambitious, they are truthful, and they are courageous. And that is precisely why they got 'ill'.

To make them believe that they are suffering from some chemical imbalance in the brain and that their recovery depends solely or even partly upon popping pills is to do them a great disfavour: it is to deny them the precious opportunity not only to identify and address important life problems, but also to develop a deeper and more refined appreciation of themselves and of the world around them—and therefore to deny them the opportunity to fulfill their highest potential as human beings.

Around the world, every mythology features a traveller who retreats, even to Hades itself in the case of Odysseus, to find himself and re-emerge as a Hero. In the *Divine Comedy*, Dante had to journey through hell and purgatory to reach the gates of heaven and find his Beatrice (Latin, 'happiness').

In the middle of our life's walk
I found myself alone in a dark forest
Where my path was confused.

Ah how hard it is to retell
How dense, dark, and dangerous
The thought of it alone fills me with fear!

So bitter than death is scarcely worse;
But to speak of the good I found there,
I shall tell of the other things that I saw.

—Dante, *The Divine Comedy, Hell*, opening verses

Chapter 4

Bipolar disorder, that fine madness

But if a man comes to the door of poetry untouched by the madness of the Muses, believing that technique alone will make him a good poet, he and his sane companions never reach perfection, but are utterly eclipsed by the performances of the inspired madman.

—Plato

Bipolar disorder, or manic-depressive illness, is a disorder of mood that involves recurrent episodes of 'mania' or 'hypo-mania' and depression. In mania and hypomania, mood is markedly elated, expansive, or irritable.

Hypomania can be thought of as a lesser degree of mania, with symptoms similar to those of mania but less severe or extreme. Mood is elated, expansive, or irritable, but, in contrast to mania, there is no marked impairment of social functioning. Hypomania may or may not herald mania.

In bipolar disorder, the frequency and severity of manic/hypomanic episodes and depressive episodes is extremely variable, as is the proportion of manic/hypomanic episodes to depressive episodes. Occasionally, episodes can be 'mixed', that is, feature symptoms of both mania and depression.

To meet the ICD-10 criteria for bipolar disorder, a person must have suffered at least two episodes of mood disturbance, at least one of which must have been mania or hypomania. To meet the DSM-5 criteria for bipolar disorder ('bipolar I disorder'), the person must have suffered at least one episode of mania. A person who has only ever suffered depressive episodes cannot be diagnosed with bipolar disorder until and unless he has also suffered a manic or hypomanic episode. In that much, mania/hypomania is the hallmark of bipolar disorder.

Since the publication of DSM-IV in 1994, DSM further distinguishes people who have suffered at least one full-blown manic episode (bipolar I disorder) from those who have only ever had one or several hypomanic episodes (bipolar II disorder). Unlike bipolar I disorder, which can be diagnosed on the basis of a single manic episode, bipolar II disorder cannot be diagnosed unless the person has also suffered at least one depressive episode.

Even so, studies indicate that a large proportion of the normal population can be found to have met the diagnostic criteria for both depression and hypomania. The concept of bipolar II disorder has been criticized, first, for lacking biological validity, even by psychiatric standards; and, second, for contributing to a false epidemic of bipolar disorder, which had hitherto been regarded as a fairly uncommon condition. This 'false epidemic' (the term is in fact that of Allen Frances, the chairman of the task force that produced DSM-IV) together with aggressive marketing by pharmaceutical companies led to many more people being prescribed potentially dangerous antipsychotic and mood stabilizing drugs.

I recall a British patient who, while studying in the US, was diagnosed with bipolar II disorder by a private psychiatrist and started on no less than four different psychotropic drugs. Upon his return to Britain, he was so drugged up that neither he nor I could distinguish symptoms from side-effects. After some debate and discussion, and a few failed attempts at reaching the private psychiatrist, we agreed to discontinue all his medication while closely monitoring his mental state. When I next saw him two weeks later, he was right back to his normal self and seemed like a much happier person. This was now several years ago, and, as far as I am aware, he has been well ever since.

DSM-IV has also been blamed for a number of other false epidemics, particularly in attention deficit hyperactivity disorder (ADHD) and Asperger's syndrome. Data from the US National Health Interview Survey indicate that, in 2012, 13.5% of boys aged 3-17 had been diagnosed with ADHD, up from 8.3% in 1997. These figures, which speak for themselves, are far higher than in the UK, partly because the ICD-10 criteria for ADHD (ICD-10: 'hyperkinetic disorder') are much more stringent. Adult ADHD, once looked upon as a rarity, is also becoming much more common, and in Canada now accounts for more than one third of all prescriptions for ADHD psycho-stimulant drugs.

First released in 2013, DSM-5 did introduce some small improvements. However, it was criticized for further narrowing the realm of normality, for instance, by dropping the 'bereavement exclusion' for depressive disorders, lowering the threshold for 'gambling disorder', and introducing such constructs as 'minor neuro-cognitive disorder', 'disruptive mood dysregulation disorder' (temper tantrums), 'premenstrual dysphoric disorder', and 'binge-eating disorder'.

Fully 69% of DSM-V task force members reported having ties to the pharmaceutical industry, up from 57% of DSM-IV task force members, raising serious questions about the soundness and integrity of the DSM revision process.

Another perhaps more fundamental issue is that classifications of mental disorders are compiled by psychiatrists who, being doctors, tend to make a false analogy between the medicine of the mind and that of the tissues. As a result, the discrete, medical-type disorders promulgated by classifications of mental disorders lack validity, and fail to map neatly onto biological findings, which, in any case, are almost entirely non-specific.

If two people with no symptoms in common can both receive the same diagnosis of schizophrenia, then what is the value of that label in describing their symptoms, deciding their treatment, or predicting their outcome, and would it not be more useful simply to describe their problems as they actually are? And if schizophrenia does not exist in nature, then how can researchers possibly find its cause or correlates? If psychiatric research has made so little progress in recent decades, it is in large part because everyone has been barking up the wrong tree. It is not a question of getting a bigger and better scanner, but of going right back to the drawing board.

What's more, medical-type labels can be as harmful as they are hollow. By reducing rich, varied, and complex human experiences to nothing more than a mental disorder, they not only sideline and trivialize those experiences but also imply an underlying defect that then serves as a pseudo-explanation for the person's disturbed behaviour. This demeans and disempowers the person, who is deterred from identifying and addressing the important life problems that underlie his distress.

In short, rather than being in any way helpful, medical-type labels actually make people worse, by perpetuating their problems, by impeding psychiatric research, and by fostering false epidemics.

People with mania frequently dress in colourful clothing or in unusual, haphazard combinations of clothing which they complement with inappropriate accessories such as hats and sunglasses and excessive make-up, jewellery, or body art. They are hyperactive, and may come across as entertaining, charming, seductive, vigilant, assertive, irritable, angry, or aggressive, and sometimes all of these in turn. Thoughts race through their mind at high speed, as a consequence of which their speech is pressured and voluble and difficult to interrupt.

In a letter to his father, a young John Ruskin (1819-1900) described the experience thus:

> *I roll on like a ball, with this exception, that contrary to the usual laws of motion I have no friction to contend with in my mind, and of course have some difficulty in stopping myself when there is nothing else to stop me ... I am almost sick and giddy with the quantity of things in my head—trains of thought beginning and branching to infinity, crossing each other, and all tempting and wanting to be worked out.*

Sometimes, the thoughts and speech of people with mania are so muddled and rambling that they are unable to stay on topic or even make a point. They may ignore the structures and strictures of grammar, step outside the confines of an English dictionary, and even talk in rhymes and puns, for example:

> *They thought I was in the pantry at home… Peekaboo… there's a magic box. Poor darling Catherine, you know, Catherine the Great, the fire grate, I'm always up the chimney. I want to scream with joy… Hallelujah!*

On top of all this, mania sufferers are typically full of grandiose or unrealistic plans and projects that they begin to act upon but then quickly abandon. They often engage in impulsive and pleasure-seeking behaviour such as spending vast amounts of money, driving recklessly, taking illegal drugs, and having sexual intercourse with near-strangers. As a result, they may end up harming themselves or others, getting into trouble with the police and other authorities, or being exploited by the less than scrupulous.

In some cases, people with mania (although not, by definition, hypomania) may experience psychotic symptoms that make their behaviour seem all the more bizarre, irrational, and chaotic. Psychotic symptoms are usually in keeping with elevated mood, and often involve delusions of grandeur, that is, delusions of exaggerated self-importance—of special status, special purpose, or special abilities. For instance, a mania sufferer may nurse the delusion that he is a brilliant scientist on the verge of discovering a cure for cancer, or that he is an exceptionally talented entrepreneur commissioned by his cousin the Queen to rid Africa of poverty.

People with mania invariably have poor insight into their mental state and find it difficult to accept that they are ill. This means that they are likely to delay and resist getting the help that they need, and, in the meantime, cause tremendous damage to their health, finances, careers, and relationships.

The case of Sophie is typical of mania and bipolar disorder:

> *Ten months ago, Sophie, a community psychiatric nurse, started feeling brighter and more energetic. At work she took on many additional roles and extra hours, but, much to her astonishment, one of her colleagues reported her as unsafe. She resigned in a fit of pique, claiming that she needed more time to devote to her other plans and projects.*
>
> *By then, she couldn't stop her thoughts from racing and was sleeping at most three or four hours a night. She bought three houses to rent out to the poor, and also leased out a launderette with the intention of converting it into a multi-purpose centre. She acted completely out of character, dressing garishly, smoking marijuana, and even getting herself arrested for brawling in the street.*
>
> *Four months ago, her mood began to drop and she felt dreadful and ashamed. Today she is feeling better but has had to sell her house to pay off her debts. Her psychiatrist suggested that she start on a mood stabilizer, but she is understandably reluctant to accept his advice.*

As aforementioned, a single episode of mania suffices to meet the DSM criteria for bipolar I disorder. The thinking behind this is that a person who has suffered a manic episode is very likely, sooner or later, to suffer one or more depressive episodes, as well as further manic or hypomanic episodes and possibly also mixed episodes.

It is important to underline that depressive episodes in bipolar disorder can be severe, with both psychotic symptoms and suicidal thoughts, as illustrated by the case of this patient, who very kindly agreed to describe his experience of suffering with bipolar disorder:

I have been high several times over the years, but low only once.

When I was high, I became very enthusiastic about some project or another and would work on it with determination and success. During such highs I wrote the bulk of two books and stood for parliament as an independent. I went to bed very late, if at all, and woke up very early. I didn't feel tired at all. There were times when I lost touch with reality and got carried away. At such times, I would jump from project to project without completing any, and did many things that I later regretted. Once I thought that I was Jesus and that I had a mission to save the world. It was an extremely alarming thought.

When I was low, I was an entirely different person. I felt as though life was pointless, with nothing worth living for. Although I would not have tried to end my life, I would not have regretted death. I did not have the wish or the energy to take on even the simplest task. Instead I spent my days sleeping or lying awake in bed, worrying about the financial problems that I created for myself during my highs. I also had a feeling of unreality, that people were conspiring to make life seem normal when in actual fact there was nothing there. I kept on asking the doctors and nurses to show me their ID because I just couldn't bring myself to believe that they were real.

Left untreated, manic episodes last for an average of about four months, and depressive episodes for an average of about six months. A bipolar sufferer can expect to suffer a total of between eight and ten episodes of mood disturbance in the course of his life, but the exact number varies a lot from person to person.

Unlike illnesses such as heart disease or diabetes, bipolar disorder tends to strike in the prime of life, when people are likely to be full of plans for the future. A person who has been freshly diagnosed with bipolar disorder may feel that all his hopes and dreams have been dashed, and that he has disappointed or even betrayed the expectations of those he holds most near and dear. Complex and often unrecognized feelings of loss, hopelessness, and guilt may exacerbate or prolong a depressive episode or give rise to further depressive episodes, and even, in some cases, to thoughts of self-harm or suicide.

It is estimated that half of bipolar sufferers attempt suicide at least once in their lifetime, and, tragically, a small number of these attempts end up being fatal. One recent Swedish study found that, compared with the normal population, suicide risk in bipolar disorder is increased 10-fold among women and 8-fold among men. Suicide risk is greatest during relapses of the illness, particularly during depressive episodes, mixed episodes, and manic episodes with psychotic symptoms. Factors likely to increase suicide risk include being male (as men have a much higher overall suicide rate), being young, lacking social support, abusing alcohol or other substances, having high ambitions or expectations, being early in the course of illness, having good insight into the illness, and having recently been discharged from a psychiatric hospital.

In addition to having a higher suicide rate, bipolar sufferers are more prone to potentially fatal accidents, particularly during manic episodes when their behaviour is rash and reckless. A person in the throes of mania is much more likely than average to be involved in a car crash, street fight, accidental drug overdose, or house fire, among others. He may also suffer from self-neglect, commonly, from forgetting or otherwise omitting to eat or drink or take his usual medication.

Life expectancy in bipolar disorder depends in large part on the course that the illness takes. Overall, life expectancy is reduced by about eight or nine years compared to average, but the gap is narrowing owing to better management, including better physical care. Perhaps surprisingly, important causes of death in bipolar disorder also include physical conditions such as cardiovascular disease, diabetes, and respiratory disease. One of the biggest contributors to poor physical health in bipolar disorder is smoking, so stopping smoking can do much to increase life expectancy, as can addressing any alcohol or drug problems, maintaining physical health through sensible diet and regular exercise, developing good sleep hygiene, avoiding stress, and seeking out early treatment for the bipolar disorder and any supervening physical conditions.

The historical terms used for the bipolar extremes both have their origins in Ancient Greek. 'Melancholy' derives from *melas* ('black') and *chole* ('bile'), because Hippocrates believed that depressed mood resulted from an excess of black bile. 'Mania' is related to *menos* ('spirit', 'force', 'passion'), *mainesthai* ('to rage', 'to go mad'), and *mantis* ('seer'), and ultimately derives from the Indo-European root *men-* ('mind'). 'Depression', a modern near synonym for melancholy, is much more recent in origin, and derives from the Latin *deprimere* ('press down', 'sink down').

The idea of a relationship between melancholy and mania can be traced back to the Ancient Greeks, and particularly to Aretaeus of Cappadocia, a physician and philosopher in the time of Nero or Vespasian. Aretaeus described a group of patients who would 'laugh, play, dance night and day, and sometimes go openly to the market crowned, as if victors in some contest of skill' only to be 'torpid, dull, and sorrowful' at other times. Although he did suggest that both patterns of behaviour resulted from one selfsame disorder, this notion did not gain currency until the industrial age.

The modern concept of bipolar disorder originated in the 19th century. In 1854, psychiatrists Jules Baillarger (1809-1890) and Jean-Pierre Falret (1794-1870) independently presented descriptions of the illness to the *Académie de Médecine* in Paris. Baillarger called it *folie à double forme* ('dual-form insanity'), whereas Falret called it *folie circulaire* ('circular insanity').

Having observed that the illness clustered in families, Falret postulated a strong genetic basis (Figure 4.1).

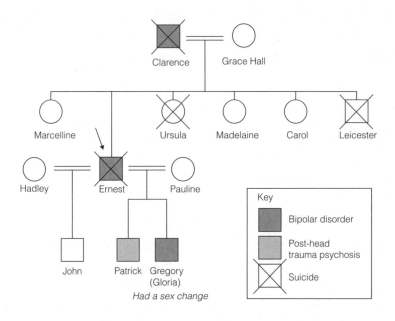

Figure 4.1. Family tree of Ernest Hemingway, who suffered from bipolar disorder. Falret correctly postulated that the illness had a strong genetic basis, stronger, in fact, than any other mental disorder. (Adapted from Jamison KR 1996.)

In the early 1900s, Kraepelin studied the natural course of the untreated illness and found it to be punctuated by relatively symptom-free intervals. On this basis, he distinguished the illness from *dementia praecox* (schizophrenia, see Chapter 2) and named it *manisch-depressives Irresein* ('manic-depressive psychosis'). He emphasized that, in contrast to *dementia praecox*, manic-depressive psychosis had an episodic course and a more benign outcome.

Interestingly, Kraepelin did not distinguish people with both manic and depressive episodes from those with only depressive episodes with psychotic symptoms. It is only in the 1950s that German psychiatrists Karl Kleist (1879-1960) and Karl Leonhard (1904-1988) proposed this divide, from which stems the contemporary emphasis on bipolarity, and hence on mania/hypomania, as the defining feature of the illness.

The term 'bipolar disorder' first appeared in the third, 1980 revision of the DSM (DSM-III). It has gradually replaced the older term 'manic-depressive illness', which, although more accurate and descriptive, did nothing to discourage people with bipolar disorder from being stigmatized as 'maniacs'.

In *Touched with Fire: Manic-Depressive Illness and the Artistic Temperament*, clinical psychologist Kay Redfield Jamison (born 1946) of John Hopkins University School of Medicine estimates that bipolar disorder is between 10 and 40 times more common among artists than in the normal population. Artists who suffered, or are thought to have suffered, from bipolar disorder include authors Hans Christian Andersen, Honoré de Balzac, F. Scott Fitzgerald, Victor Hugo, Edgar Allan Poe, Mary Shelley, Mark Twain, and Virginia Woolf; poets William Blake, John Clare, TS Eliot,

Florbela Espanca, John Keats, Robert Lowell, Fernando Pessoa, Alfred Lord Tennyson, and Walt Whitman; and composers Ludwig van Beethoven, Hector Berlioz, Edward Elgar, George Frederic Handel, Gustav Mahler, Sergei Rachmaninoff, Robert Schumann, and Peter Tchaikovsky—to name but a handful.

Some of these artists went so far as to credit their creative genius with their 'moods of the mind'.

For instance, Edgar Allan Poe (1809-1849) had the narrator of his semi-autobiographical short story *Eleonora* relate:

> *I am come of a race noted for vigor of fancy and ardour of passion. Men have called me mad; but the question is not yet settled, whether madness is or is not the loftiest intelligence—whether much that is glorious—whether all that is profound—does not spring from disease of thought—from moods of mind exalted at the expense of the general intellect. They who dream by day are cognizant of many things which escape those who dream only by night. In their gray visions they obtain glimpses of eternity, and thrill, in awakening, to find that they have been upon the verge of the great secret. In snatches, they learn something of the wisdom which is of good, and more of the knowledge which is of evil. They penetrate, however rudderless or compassless, into the vast ocean of the 'light ineffable'...*

Poe's poem *The Raven* speaks of the mysterious visit of a talking raven to a distraught lover on the brink of madness. The poem is famous for its musicality, stylized language, and supernatural atmosphere, and it is possible that the raven represents either Poe's mental disorder or his related alcoholism.

In the final stanza, Poe alludes to Pallas Athena, the Greek goddess of wisdom:

> *And the Raven, never flitting, still is sitting, still is sitting*
> *On the pallid bust of Pallas just above my chamber door;*
> *And his eyes have all the seeming of a demon's that is dreaming,*
> *And the lamplight o'er him streaming throws his shadow on the floor;*
> *And my soul from out that shadow that lies floating on the floor*
> *Shall be lifted—nevermore!*

Virginia Woolf (1882-1941) suffered from bipolar disorder from the age of 13. At the age of 59, she committed suicide by walking into the River Ouse with a large rock in her pocket. This final episode of her life is memorably portrayed in *The Hours*, a film loosely based on the novel *Mrs Dalloway* and starring Nicole Kidman as Virginia Woolf.

In *Mrs Dalloway*, Woolf writes of her alter ego Dalloway:

> *She felt very young; at the same time unspeakably aged. She sliced*
> *like a knife through everything; at the same time was outside,*
> *looking on… far out to sea and alone; she always had the feeling*
> *that it was very, very dangerous to live even one day.*

Woolf wrote of her own mental illness in a letter to her friend Ethel Smyth:

> *I married, and then my brains went up like a shower of fireworks.*
> *As an experience, madness is terrific I can assure you, and not to*
> *be sniffed at; and in its lava I still find most of the things that I*
> *write about. It shoots out of one everything shaped, final, not in*
> *mere driblets as sanity does. And the six months… that I lay in bed*
> *taught me a good deal about what is called oneself.*

In the 1970s, psychiatrist Nancy Andreasen (born 1938) carried out the first empirical study of mental disorder and creativity. She studied the medical histories of a group of 30 prominent authors associated with the Iowa Writers' Workshop (including Kurt Vonnegut, Richard Yates, and John Cheever), expecting to reveal a relationship between creativity and schizophrenia in close relatives. In the event, she found no such relationship, but did uncover a strong correlation between creativity and mood disorders. Fully 80 per cent of the authors in her sample had experienced at least one episode of major depression, hypomania, or mania, compared to only 30 per cent of a matched control group. Prof Andreasen decided to follow up on her authors over the next 15 years. After the 15 years, 43% of the authors met the criteria for bipolar disorder, compared to only 10 per cent of the control group and 1 per cent of the general population. Tragically, two of the authors—out of just 30—had committed suicide. For Prof Andreasen, 'Issues of statistical significance pale before the clinical implications of this fact.'

In 1989, inspired by the findings of the Iowa Writers' Workshop study, Prof Jamison surveyed 47 British authors and visual artists from the British Royal Academy. She found that 38 per cent of her sample had received treatment for a mood disorder, including over half of the playwrights and poets. Responding to questions about the role of very intense moods in the creative process, many authors and artists in the sample reported changes in mood, cognition, and behaviour, either preceding or coinciding with creative episodes. They described 'increases in enthusiasm, energy, self-confidence, speed of mental association, fluency of thoughts and elevated mood, and a strong sense of well-being'—all features which overlap with the symptoms of hypomania.

Unusually among mental or indeed physical disorders, bipolar disorder is *more* common in higher socioeconomics groups, suggesting that the genes that predispose to bipolar disorder also predispose to greater achievement and success in the relatives of bipolar sufferers and perhaps even in bipolar sufferers themselves. A prime example is Prof Jamison herself, who is not only Professor of Psychiatry but also Honorary Professor of English. Jamison has written a number of critically acclaimed books, including one, called *An Unquiet Mind*, on her experience of suffering with bipolar disorder.

While the genes responsible for bipolar disorder may lead to adaptive advantages at the level of the individual, they may also lead to adaptive advantages at the level of the tribe or group. Compared to neighbouring population groups, population groups with a higher proportion of creative individuals are likely to be more artistically and culturally developed, with a stronger sense of identity and purpose and tighter social cohesion. They are also likely to be more technologically advanced, and so more economically and militarily successful. Owing to these important adaptive advantages, population groups with a higher proportion of creative individuals stand a better chance of surviving and flourishing, and, with them, the genes for bipolar disorder.

The risk of a first-degree relative of a bipolar sufferer also developing bipolar disorder is about 9 per cent. As well as bipolar disorder, first-degree relatives of bipolar sufferers are at increased risk of unipolar depression and 'schizoaffective disorder', which is a condition characterized by prominent affective *and* schizophrenic symptoms in the same episode of illness. This supports the hypothesis that schizophrenia and affective disorders such as bipolar disorder lie, contra Kraepelin, on a single spectrum of psychotic disorders, with schizoaffective disorder in the middle of the spectrum.

Moreover, there is mounting evidence that bipolar disorder and schizophrenia share some of the same genetic determinants, and that these overlapping sets of genes both predispose to greater creativity through loosened associations or so-called divergent thinking. As Nietzsche remarked in *Thus Spoke Zarathustra*, 'One must have chaos in one, to give birth to a dancing star.'

It is often assumed that a highly creative person is also a highly intelligent one, and so the question naturally arises as to whether intelligence and creativity reflect one and the same construct. A majority of studies examining correlations between intelligence and creativity suggest that they do not. For instance, in the Iowa Writers' Workshop study, the average IQ of the prominent authors was 'only' 120, and no higher than the average IQ of the 'non-creative' matched control group.

According to the 'threshold hypothesis' proposed by psychologist Ellis Paul Torrance (1915-2003), high intelligence is a necessary but insufficient condition for high creativity. In other words, while all highly creative people are highly intelligent, not all highly intelligent people are highly creative, with other determinants such as personality or temperament coming into play.

An alternative hypothesis is that high intelligence and high creativity both arise from the selfsame cognitive processes; whereas intelligence is assessed more in terms of the presence of these cognitive processes, creativity is assessed more in terms of their worthwhile application. If this alternative hypothesis is correct, then the genes that predispose to mental disorder and creativity might also predispose to intelligence.

For Prof Andreasen, creative people stand apart from the slumbering masses in being more open to ideas and experiences and more tolerant of ambiguity. Such traits enable them to see and feel and understand more, but they also expose them to doubt, rejection, and dark moods. A creative person experiences the order and structure that others take for granted as inhibiting, even suffocating. So he feels the need to confront norms and conventions, discard the certitudes of black and white definition, and escape into a richer and subtler 'borderless grey'. The freedom that he discovers in this limbo allows him to enter into states of intense focus and concentration marked by heightened consciousness, supercharged activity, and intense productivity. Such states, which are akin to hypomania, are the hallmark of the creative process.

In a letter to his patron Nadezhda von Meck, Peter Tchaikovsky (1840-1893) described the experience thus:

> *It would be in vain to try to put into words, that immeasurable sense of bliss which comes over me directly as a new idea awakens in me and begins to assume a definite form. I forget everything and behave like a madman. Everything within me starts pulsing and quivering; hardly have I begun the sketch ere one thought follows another. In the midst of this magic process it frequently happens that some external interruption wakes me from my somnambulistic state… Dreadful, indeed, are such interruptions.*

In Plato's *Ion*, on the subject of inspiration, Socrates tells Ion, a prize-winning rhapsode (performer of epic poetry) from Ephesus, that:

> *…the poet is a light and winged and holy thing, and there is no invention in him until he has been inspired and is out of his senses, and the mind is no longer in him: when he has not attained to this state, he is powerless and is unable to utter his oracles.*

After carrying out a detailed study of some of the most eminent personalities of the 20th century, psychiatrist Felix Post (1913-2001) postulated that the psychological discomfort that accompanies a mental disorder can in itself be an important driver of creative expression, and many writers and artists have asserted that the creative act enables them both to stave off and to sublimate their depressive anguish.

As psychiatrist Anthony Storr (1920-2001) remarked in his inspired book on solitude:

> *The creative process can be a way of protecting the individual against being overwhelmed by depression, a means of regaining a sense of mastery in those who have lost it, and, to a varying extent, a way of repairing the self damaged by bereavement or by the loss of confidence in human relationships which accompanies depression from whatever cause.*

A 2007 study by Santosa and colleagues found that bipolar sufferers and creative discipline controls scored significantly higher than healthy controls on a measure of creativity called the Barron-Welsh Art Scale. In a related study, the researchers sought to identify temperamental traits that bipolar sufferers and highly creative people have in common. They found that both shared tendencies for mild elation and depression with gradual shifts from the one to the other, openness, irritability, and neuroticism (roughly speaking, a combination of anxiety and perfectionism). During periods of mild depression, bipolar sufferers and creative people may be able to retreat inside themselves, introspect, put thoughts and feelings into perspective, eliminate irrelevant ideas, and focus on bare essentials. Later, during periods of mild elation, they may be able to gather the vision, confidence, and stamina for creative expression and realization.

Shifts in mood may be evidenced in the creative acts of bipolar sufferers, for example, in the compositions of Tchaikovsky, particularly the crypto-biographical *Swan Lake*. Yet it must be stressed, first, that not all bipolar sufferers are creative, and, second, that even those who are tend to peak during periods of remission when symptoms are either mild or absent. Most creative bipolar sufferers cannot create when depressed, but instead use their depression as a source of inspiration for their next piece of work; nor can they create when manic or psychotic because their concentration is too poor and their thinking too disorganized to produce anything substantial or coherent.

Many creative genii are not bipolar sufferers; conversely, most bipolar sufferers are not creative genii. Thus, bipolar disorder is neither necessary nor sufficient for creative genius. As there are fewer bipolar sufferers who are artists than artists who are bipolar sufferers, one could argue that it is in fact creative genius that predisposes to bipolar disorder. And while bipolar sufferers may indeed be more creative than average, this might simply reflect a well-documented propensity in bipolar sufferers to pursue careers in the arts. No one can doubt that bipolar disorder and creative genius are associated, but correlation is not causation, and, to critics, evidence of causation and of the direction of causation is still lacking. As Prof Andreasen recently wrote, 'The study of the relationship between creativity and mental illnesses is still a relatively open territory, with much remaining to be done.'

Even though the modern concept of bipolar disorder originated in the 19th century, the first effective treatments for the illness did not appear until the second half of the 20th century. The Australian psychiatrist and researcher John Cade (1912-1980) serendipitously discovered the mood stabilizing properties of lithium in 1949, but the naturally occurring salt took another two decades to enter into mainstream practice.

Today, the choice of medication in bipolar disorder is largely determined by the person's symptoms. In a manic episode, the treatment most often prescribed is an antipsychotic; in a depressive episode, it is an antidepressant, sometimes in conjunction with an antipsychotic to avoid 'manic switch' (that is, over-treatment into mania). Rarely, ECT might be prescribed, either for a depressive episode that has become threatening or unresponsive, or, even more rarely, for a manic episode that cannot be treated with medication, either because it is unresponsive to medication or because medication is contraindicated. Once symptoms of mania or depression have remitted, the antipsychotic or antidepressant is usually discontinued and replaced with a mood stabilizer such as lithium or the anticonvulsant valproate to reduce the risk of further relapses into mania and depression.

Lithium is often said to decrease the rate of relapse by about one-third, and to be more effective against mania than depression. Its mode of action is unclear, but it is held to have a range of effects in the brain, including on certain neurotransmitters and their receptors.

Understandably, many bipolar sufferers are reluctant to start on lithium owing to the complexities and risks involved. In particular, some bipolar sufferers who value or depend upon their creativity fear that the drug may leave them unable to think, feel, and work.

As poet Rainer Maria Rilke (1875-1926) put it, 'If my devils were to leave me, I am afraid my angels will take flight as well.'

The other side of the argument is that, by reducing the risk of relapse, lithium can actually enable bipolar sufferers to create much more. After the advent of lithium, poet Robert Lowell (1917-1977) is reported to have said, 'I'm doing so much better. I'm so much more productive… My problem was a deficiency in salt. And now that I'm taking this lithium salt, I'm very stable.'

Ideally, lithium should only be started if there is a clear intention to carry on with it for at least three years, as poor compliance and intermittent treatment may precipitate episodes of 'rebound' mania and hypomania. The serum level of lithium needs to be within a narrow range, or 'therapeutic window', of about 0.5-1.0 millimoles per litre: any less and the beneficial effects are limited, any more and side- and toxic effects become much likelier. For the person starting on lithium, this means frequent blood tests until the serum level is in range.

Short-term side-effects of lithium include a stuffy nose and metallic taste in the mouth, confusion, fine tremor, nausea, diarrhoea, muscle weakness, and increased thirst and urination. In the longer term, lithium can cause swelling and weight gain and make certain skin conditions such as acne and psoriasis flare up. As lithium can damage the thyroid gland and kidneys, thyroid and kidney function must be monitored at regular intervals, along with serum levels. Lithium can also affect the conduction of electrical impulses in the heart, and it is standard practice to record a tracing of the heart (an ECG) prior to starting treatment.

High serum lithium levels give rise to additional toxic effects, among which anorexia, nausea, vomiting, diarrhoea, coarse tremor, difficulty articulating speech, clumsiness, unsteadiness, and, in severe cases, fits and loss of consciousness. People on lithium need to drink plenty of fluids and keep up their salt intake, as dehydration and salt depletion can increase serum levels and lead to lithium toxicity.

Given all these hazards and hurdles, many bipolar sufferers delay starting on lithium until after they have suffered from one or more further relapses, or else carefully consider other options such as valproate or an antipsychotic drug, which, of course, have drawbacks of their own.

Joanna Moncrieff, a psychiatrist, researcher, and co-chair of the Critical Psychiatry Network, argues that the evidence for the effectiveness of lithium in the treatment of bipolar disorder is 'far too weak to outweigh the harm it can cause'. According to Dr Moncrieff, the main problem with the evidence for lithium is that the higher rate of relapse in control groups is in fact artificial. In every randomized trial looking at lithium, at least some of the people in the control group withdrew from lithium to start on a placebo, and there is substantial evidence that withdrawing from lithium can precipitate a relapse or 'rebound', especially in mania or hypomania. Even if lithium could be shown to reduce relapse rates, says Dr Moncrieff, this would owe more to its sedating and slowing effects than to any specific mood stabilizing effect. Moreover, the sudden removal of this neurological suppression could be responsible for the rebound phenomenon.

Yet, lithium also has it supporters, not least Prof Jamison herself. In *An Unquiet Mind*, she confides:

I have often asked myself whether, given the choice, I would choose to have manic-depressive illness. If lithium were not available to me, or didn't work for me, the answer would be a simple no … and it would be an answer laced with terror. But lithium does work for me, and therefore I can afford to pose the question. Strangely enough, I think I would choose to have it. It's complicated… Depression is awful beyond words or sounds or images … So why would I want anything to do with this illness? Because I honestly believe that as a result of it I have felt more things, more deeply; had more experiences, more intensely; loved more, and have been more loved; laughed more often for having cried more often; appreciated more the springs, for all the winters… Depressed, I have crawled on my hands and knees in order to get across a room and have done it for month after month. But normal or manic I have run faster, thought faster, and loved faster than most I know. And I think much of this is related to my illness—the intensity it gives to things.

Chapter 5

Anxiety, freedom, and death

Anxiety is the dizziness of freedom.

—Søren Kierkegaard

On October 30, 1938, Orson Welles (1915-1985) broadcast an episode of the radio drama *Mercury Theatre on the Air*. This episode, entitled *The War of the Worlds* and based on a novel by HG Wells (1866-1946), suggested to listeners that a Martian invasion was taking place. In the charged atmosphere of the days leading up to the Second World War, many people missed or ignored the opening credits and mistook the radio drama for a news broadcast. Panic ensued and people began to flee, with some even reporting flashes of light and a smell of poison gas (Figure 5.1).

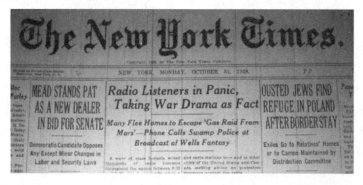

Figure 5.1. New York Times headlines on October 31, 1938. 'Radio Listeners in Panic, Taking War Drama as Fact.'

This panic, a form of mass hysteria, is one of the many forms that anxiety can take. But what is anxiety, what purpose does it serve, and when does it become a problem?

Anxiety can be defined as 'a state consisting of psychological and physical symptoms brought about by a sense of apprehension at a perceived threat'. Fear is similar to anxiety, except that with fear the threat is, or is perceived to be, more concrete, present, or imminent.

The psychological and physical symptoms of anxiety vary according to the nature and magnitude of the perceived threat, and from one person to another. Psychological symptoms may include feelings of fear and dread, an exaggerated startle reflex, poor concentration, irritability, and insomnia. In mild to moderate anxiety, physical symptoms such as tremor, sweating, muscle tension, a faster heart rate, and faster and deeper breathing arise from the body's so-called fight-or-flight response, a state of high arousal fuelled by a surge in adrenaline. Some people can also develop a dry mouth together with the irritating feeling of having a lump in the throat. This feeling, referred to in the medical jargon as *globus hystericus*, is associated with forced swallowing and a characteristic gulping sound that is often exploited in children's cartoons to signal fear.

In severe anxiety, over-breathing (hyperventilation) can lead to a fall in the concentration of carbon dioxide in the blood. This gives rise to an additional set of physical symptoms, among which chest discomfort, numbness or tingling in the hands and feet, dizziness, and faintness.

Some children play a dangerous game in which they hyperventilate and then perform the Valsalva manoeuvre to make themselves faint. The Valsalva manoeuvre involves placing a thumb in the mouth and blowing hard against it, without releasing any air. This increases the pressure in the thoracic cavity, impeding the return of venous blood to the heart and precipitating a rapid drop in blood pressure.

Fear and anxiety can be a normal response to life experiences, a protective mechanism that has evolved both to prevent us from entering into potentially dangerous situations and to assist us in escaping from them should they befall us regardless. For instance, anxiety can prevent us from coming into close contact with disease-carrying or poisonous animals such as rats, snakes, and spiders; from engaging with a much stronger or angrier enemy; and even from declaring our undying love to someone who is unlikely to spare our feelings. If we do find ourselves in a potentially dangerous situation, the fight-or-flight response triggered by fear can help us to mount an appropriate response by priming our body for action and increasing our performance and stamina.

In short, the purpose of fear and anxiety is to preserve us from harm, and, above all, from death—whether it be literal or metaphorical, biological or psychosocial.

Although some degree of anxiety can improve our performance on a range of tasks, severe or inappropriate anxiety can have the opposite effect and hinder our performance. Thus, whereas a confident actor may perform optimally in front of a live audience, a novice may suffer from stage fright and freeze. The relationship between anxiety and performance can be expressed graphically by a parabola or inverted 'U' (Figure 5.2).

According to the Yerkes-Dodson curve, our performance increases with arousal but only up to a certain point, beyond which it starts to decline. The Yerkes-Dodson curve best applies to complex or difficult tasks, rather than simple tasks for which the relationship between arousal and performance is more linear.

Also important is the nature of the task. Generally speaking, intellectual challenges require a lower level of arousal for optimal performance than tasks that call for strength and stamina. This makes good sense, since those situations that trigger the greatest anxiety are generally those that call for the greatest strength and stamina, for instance, to face a foe or scamper up the nearest tree.

The Yerkes-Dodson curve indicates that very high levels of anxiety can result in handicap, even paralysis. From a medical standpoint,

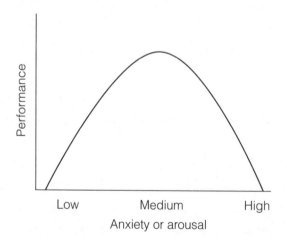

Figure 5.2. The Yerkes-Dodson curve is named after psychologists RM Yerkes and JD Dodson.

anxiety becomes problematic when it becomes so severe, frequent, or longstanding as to prevent us from fulfilling our occupational or social obligations. This often owes to a primary anxiety disorder, although in some instances the anxiety is secondary to another psychiatric disorder such as depression or schizophrenia, or to a medical disorder such as hyperthyroidism or alcohol withdrawal. Primary anxiety disorders are very common, affecting almost one in every five people in the US in any given year. As broadly conceived, they present in a variety of forms, including phobic anxiety disorders, panic disorder, generalized anxiety disorder, conversion disorders, post-traumatic stress disorder, and culture-bound syndromes.

Phobic anxiety disorders are the most common type of anxiety disorder, and involve the persistent and irrational fear of an object, activity, or situation. DSM-V and ICD-10 recognize three types of phobic anxiety disorder: agoraphobia, social phobia, and specific phobia.

The term 'agoraphobia' derives from the Greek *phobos* ('fear') and *agora* ('market', 'marketplace'), and so literally means 'fear of the marketplace'. Contrary to popular belief, agoraphobia does not describe a fear of open spaces, but a fear of places that are difficult or embarrassing to escape from, typically because they are confined, crowded, or far from home. In time, people with agoraphobia may become increasingly homebound, and reliant on one or more trusted companions to accompany them on their outings.

Interestingly, there seems to be an association between agoraphobia and poor spatial orientation, suggesting that spatial disorientation, particularly in places where visual cues are sparse, may contribute to the development of the disorder. Spatial orientation is critical from an evolutionary standpoint, since it enables us not only to locate ourselves, but also our friends and foes, sources of food and water, and places of shelter and safety.

Social phobia is the fear of being judged by others and of being embarrassed or humiliated in one or more social or performance situations such as holding a conversation or delivering a speech.

The problem is not new, and Hippocrates himself once described someone who:

> ...*through bashfulness, suspicion, and timorousness, will not be seen abroad; loves darkness as life and cannot endure the light or to sit in lightsome places; his hat still in his eyes, he will neither see, nor be seen by his good will. He dare not come in company for fear he should be misused, disgraced, overshoot himself in gesture or speeches, or be sick; he thinks every man observes him.*

Social phobia (DSM-5: social anxiety disorder) has many features in common with shyness, and distinguishing between the two can be a cause for debate and controversy. Some critics claim that the label is no more than an attempt to pass off a problematic personality trait as a mental disorder and thereby to legitimize its medical 'treatment'. Proponents retort that social phobia differs from simple shyness in that it usually starts at a later age and is more severe and debilitating, with much more prominent anxiety. In addition, whereas social phobia is invariably maladaptive, a certain degree of shyness can be adaptive in so far as it can protect our self-esteem and social standing, and preserve us from interacting too closely with potentially hostile or abusive strangers—which is no doubt why shyness is most pronounced in children and other vulnerable groups.

Specific phobia is by far the most common of the three phobic anxiety disorders. As its name implies, it is the fear of a specific object, activity, or situation. Common specific phobias include arachnophobia (spiders), acrophobia (heights), claustrophobia (enclosed spaces), achluophobia (darkness), brontophobia (storms), and haematophobia (blood). Unlike other anxiety disorders, which tend to begin in adulthood, specific phobias often trace their beginnings to early childhood. Moreover, we seem to have a strong innate predisposition for phobias of the natural dangers commonly faced by our ancestors such as spiders and heights, even if manmade hazards such as motor vehicles, electric cables, and text messaging now pose much greater threats to our chances of surviving and reproducing.

In a phobic anxiety disorder (whether agoraphobia, social phobia, or a specific phobia), exposure to the feared object, activity, or situation can trigger an attack of severe anxiety, or panic attack. During a panic attack, symptoms of anxiety are so severe that the person fears that he is suffocating, having a heart attack, losing control, or even 'going crazy'. In time, he comes to develop a fear of the panic attacks themselves, which in turn sets off further panic attacks. A vicious circle takes hold, with the panic attacks becoming ever more frequent and ever more severe and even occurring 'out of the blue'.

This pattern of recurrent panic attacks, which is referred to as 'panic disorder', can superimpose itself onto any anxiety disorder as well as depression, substance misuse, and certain physical conditions such as hyperthyroidism. Panic disorder often leads to so-called secondary agoraphobia, in which the person becomes increasingly homebound so as to minimize the risk and consequences of suffering further panic attacks.

Anxiety disorders need not be specifically directed as in phobic anxiety disorders. In generalized anxiety disorder (GAD), anxiety is not directed at any particular object, activity, or situation, but is free-floating and far-reaching. There is apprehension about a number of hypothetical events that is completely out of proportion to the actual likelihood or potential impact of those events. People with GAD fear the future to such an extent that they behave in a manner that is overly cautious and risk-averse. They are, quite literally, 'paralyzed with fear'.

After a traumatic event such as a physical or sexual assault, anxiety may be so sudden and overwhelming that it cannot be processed. As a result, the anxiety is converted into other symptoms such as limb paralysis, speech loss, or blindness. This 'conversion disorder' may be accompanied by loss of memory for the traumatic event, and the person might even depart on a sudden and unexpected journey. During this journey, or 'dissociative fugue', the person is typically confused about his personal identity, and may even take on a separate identity. Compared to conversion disorder, dissociative fugue is rare.

Another form of dissociative disorder is possession trance, in which the person reacts to trauma by adopting another identity, commonly that of a ghost, spirit, or deity. In many cultures, a trance is an accepted and even exalted expression of religious feeling, and should only be considered problematic or potentially problematic if it is completely out of keeping with the person's culture or sub-culture.

Anxiety related to a traumatic event can also manifest in the form of post-traumatic stress disorder (PTSD). This condition was first recognized in the aftermath of the First World War, and its historical epithets include 'shell shock', 'combat neurosis', and 'survivor syndrome'. Common symptoms of PTSD include anxiety, of course, but also numbing, detachment, flashbacks, nightmares, partial or complete amnesia for the traumatic event, and avoidance of reminders of the traumatic event—although not all of these symptoms need to be present for a diagnosis to be made. The symptoms can last for several years, and predispose to secondary mental disorders such as depression, other anxiety disorders, and alcohol and drug misuse.

Generally speaking, culture-specific, or culture-bound, syndromes are mental disturbances that only find expression in certain cultures or ethnic groups, and that are not comfortably accommodated by Western psychiatric classifications. DSM-IV defined them as 'recurrent, locality-specific patterns of aberrant behavior and troubling experience…'

One example of a culture-bound syndrome is dhat, which is seen in men from South Asia, and involves sudden anxiety about loss of semen in the urine, whitish discoloration of the urine, and sexual dysfunction, combined with feelings of weakness and exhaustion. The syndrome may originate in the Hindu belief that it takes forty drops of blood to create a drop of bone marrow, and forty drops of bone marrow to create a drop of semen, and thus that semen is a concentrated essence of life.

DSM-5 replaces the notion of culture-bound syndromes with three 'cultural concepts of distress': cultural syndromes, cultural idioms of distress, and cultural explanations for distress. Rather than merely listing specific cultural syndromes, DSM-5 adopts a broader approach to cultural issues, and acknowledges that all mental disorders, including DSM disorders, can be culturally shaped.

However, some DSM disorders are, it seems, much more culturally shaped than others. For instance, PTSD, anorexia nervosa, bulimia nervosa, depression, and deliberate self-harm (non-suicidal self-injury) can all be understood as cultural syndromes. Yet, for being in the DSM, they are usually seen, and largely legitimized, as biological and therefore universal expressions of human distress.

Thus, a further criticism of classifications of mental disorders such as DSM and ICD is that, arm in arm with pharmaceutical companies, they encourage the wholesale exportation of Western mental disorders, and, more than that, the wholesale exportation of Western accounts of mental disorder, Western approaches to mental disorder, and, ultimately, Western values such as biologism, individualism, and the medicalization of distress and deviance.

In her recent book, *Depression in Japan*, anthropologist Junko Kitanaka writes that, until relatively recently, depression (*utsubyō*) had remained largely unknown to the lay population of Japan. Between 1999 and 2008, the number of people diagnosed with depression more than doubled as psychiatrists and pharmaceutical companies urged people to re-interpret their distress in terms of depression. Depression, says Kitanaka, is now one of the most frequently cited reasons for taking sick leave, and has been 'transformed from a rare disease to one of the most talked about illnesses in recent Japanese history'.

In *Crazy Like Us: The Globalization of the American Psyche*, journalist Ethan Watters shows how psychiatric imperialism is leading to a pandemic of Western disease categories and treatments. Watters argues that changing a culture's ideas about mental disorder actually changes that culture's disorders, and depletes the store of local beliefs and customs which, in many cases, provided better answers to people's problems than antidepressants and anti-psychotics. For Watters, the most devastating consequence of our impact on other cultures is not our golden arches, but the bulldozing of the human psyche itself.

He writes:

> *Looking at ourselves through the eyes of those living in places where human tragedy is still embedded in complex religious and cultural narratives, we get a glimpse of our modern selves as a deeply insecure and fearful people. We are investing our great wealth in researching and treating this disorder because we have rather suddenly lost other belief systems that once gave meaning and context to our suffering.*

Distressed people are subconsciously driven to externalize their suffering, partly to make it more manageable, and partly so that it can be recognized and legitimized. According to medical historian Edward Shorter, our culture's beliefs and narratives about illness provide us with a limited number of templates or models of illness by which to externalize our distress. If authorities such as psychiatrists and celebrities appear to endorse or condone a new template such as ADHD or deliberate self-harm, the template enters into our culture's 'symptom pool' and the condition starts to spread. At the same time, tired templates seep out of the symptom pool, which may explain why conditions such as 'hysteria' and catatonic schizophrenia (schizophrenia dominated by extreme agitation or immobility and odd mannerisms and posturing) have become so rare.

The incidence of bulimia nervosa rose in 1992, the year in which journalist Andrew Morton exposed Princess Diana's 'secret disease', and peaked in 1995, when she revealed her eating disorder to the public. It began to decline in 1997, the year of her tragic death. This synchronology suggests that Princess Diana's status and glamour combined with intense press coverage of her bulimia and bulimia in general led to an increase in the incidence of the disorder.

An alternative explanation is that Princess Diana's example encouraged people to come forward and admit to their eating disorder. By the same token, it could have been that the Japanese had always suffered from depression, but had been hiding it, or had not had a template by which to recognize or externalize it. The danger for us psychiatrists and health professionals when treating people with mental disorder is to treat the template without addressing or even acknowledging the very real distress that lies beneath.

Returning more specifically to the subject of anxiety, the Orson Welles broadcast of October 30, 1938 is evidence enough that mass hysteria can befall us at any time. In 1989, 150 children took part in a summer programme at a youth centre in Florida. Each day at noon, the children gathered in the dining hall to be served pre-packed lunches. One day, a girl complained that her sandwich did not taste right. She felt nauseated, went to the toilet, and returned saying that she had vomited. Almost immediately, other children began experiencing symptoms such as nausea, abdominal cramps, and tingling in the hands and feet. The supervisor asked the children to stop eating for fear that the food was poisoned. Within 40 minutes, 63 children were sick and more than 25 had vomited.

The children were sent to one of three hospitals, but every test performed turned out to be negative, as did meal sample analyses for pathogens and poisons. Food processing and storing standards had been scrupulously observed, and no illness had been reported from any of the other 68 sites at which the pre-packed lunches had been served.

As with the Orson Welles broadcast, a tense atmosphere had been created by the revelation two days earlier of management problems at the youth centre. The children had no doubt picked up on the staff's anxiety, which had made them more suggestible to the first girl's complaints. After the supervisor, a figure of authority, had announced that the food may be poisoned, the situation simply spiraled out of control.

Although mass hysteria itself is relatively uncommon, cases such as these do call attention to our propensity to somatize, that is, to convert our anxiety and distress into more concrete physical symptoms. Somatization, which can be thought of as an ego defence, is an unconscious process, and people who somatize do not usually recognize the psychological origins of their symptoms. To them, their symptoms are entirely real, and they are also entirely real in the important sense that, despite their psychological origins, they do actually exist: the limb cannot move, the eye cannot see, and so on. The tendency to concretize psychic pain is deeply ingrained in our human nature, and should not be confused or even amalgamated with a factitious disorder or malingering.

In recent decades, it has become increasingly apparent that psychological stressors can lead to physical symptoms not only through somatization but also by physical processes involving the nervous, endocrine, and immune systems. For instance, one recent study conducted by Dr Elizabeth Mostofsky of Harvard Medical School found that the first 24 hours of bereavement are associated with a staggering 21-fold increase in the risk of heart attack.

Since the initial experiments of psychologist Robert Ader (1932-2011) on lab rats in the 1970s, the field of psychoneuroimmunology has truly blossomed. The large and ever increasing body of evidence that it continues to uncover has led to the mainstream recognition not only of the adverse effects of psychological stress on health, recovery, and ageing, but also of the beneficial effects of positive emotions such as tranquility, motivation, and a sense of purpose or meaning.

Here again, modern science has barely caught up with the wisdom of the ancients, who were well aware of the strong links between psychological and physical health. In the *Charmides*, one of Plato's early dialogues, Socrates tells the young Charmides, who has been suffering from headaches, about a charm for headaches which he learnt from one of the mystical physicians to the king of Thrace. However, this great physician taught that it is best to cure the soul before curing the body, since health and happiness ultimately depend on the state of the soul.

> *He said all things, both good and bad, in the body and in the whole man, originated in the soul and spread from there… One ought, then, to treat the soul first and foremost, if the head and the rest of the body were to be well. He said the soul was treated with certain charms, my dear Charmides, and that these charms were beautiful words. As a result of such words self-control came into being in souls. When it came into being and was present in them, it was then easy to secure health both for the head and for the rest of the body.*

People with a high level of anxiety have historically been referred to as 'neurotic'. The term 'neurosis' derives from the Ancient Greek *neuron* ('nerve'), and loosely means 'disease of the nerves'. The core feature of neurosis is a high level of 'background' anxiety, but neurosis can also manifest in the form of other symptoms such as phobias, panic attacks, irritability, perfectionism, and obsessive-compulsive tendencies. Although very common in some form or other, neurosis can prevent us from living in the moment, adapting usefully to our environment, and developing a richer, more complex, and more fulfilling outlook on life.

Carl Jung believed that neurotic people fundamentally had issues with the purpose and meaning of their life. In his autobiography of 1961, *Memories, Dreams, Reflections*, he noted that the majority of his patients 'consisted not of believers but of those who had lost their faith'. Interestingly, Jung also believed that neurosis could be beneficial to some people despite its debilitating effects.

In *Two Essays on Analytical Psychology*, he wrote:

> *The reader will doubtless ask: What in the world is the value and*
> *meaning of a neurosis, this most useless and pestilent curse*
> *of humanity? To be neurotic—what good can that do? ... I*
> *myself have known more than one person who owed his whole*
> *usefulness and reason for existence to a neurosis, which prevented*
> *all the worst follies in his life and forced him to a mode of living*
> *that developed his valuable potentialities. These might have been*
> *stifled had not the neurosis, with iron grip, held him to the place*
> *where he belonged.*

The most original, influential, and polemical theory of the origins of neurosis is that of Sigmund Freud. Freud studied medicine at the University of Vienna from 1873 to 1881, and, after some time, decided to specialize in neurology. In 1885-86, he spent the best part of a year in Paris, and returned to Vienna inspired by neurologist Jean-Martin Charcot's use of hypnosis in the treatment of 'hysteria', an outdated construct involving the conversion of anxiety into physical and psychological symptoms. Freud opened a private practice for the treatment of neuropsychiatric disorders, but eventually abandoned hypnosis for 'free association', which involves asking the patient to relax on a couch and say whatever comes into her mind (Freud's patients were mostly women). In 1895, inspired by the case of a patient called Bertha Pappenheim ('Anna O.'), Freud published the seminal *Studies on Hysteria* with his friend and colleague Josef Breuer. Following the public successes of *The Interpretation of Dreams* (1899) and *The Psychopathology of Everyday Life* (1901), he obtained a professorship at the University of Vienna and began to gather a devoted following. He remained a prolific writer throughout his life. Some of his most important works include *Three Essays on the Theory of Sexuality* (1905), *Totem and Taboo* (1913), and *Beyond the Pleasure Principle* (1920). Following the Nazi annexation of Austria in 1938, he fled to London, where, in the following year, he died of cancer of the jaw.

In *Studies on Hysteria*, Freud and Breuer formulated the psycho-analytic theory according to which neuroses have their origins in deeply traumatic and consequently repressed experiences. Treatment requires the patient to recall these repressed experiences into consciousness and to confront them once and for all, leading to a sudden and dramatic outpouring of emotion ('catharsis') and the gaining of insight. Such outcomes can be achieved through the methods of free association and dream interpretation, and by a sort of passivity on the part of the psychoanalyst. This passivity transforms the analyst into a blank canvas onto which the patient can unconsciously project her thoughts and feelings ('transference'). At the same time, the analyst should guard against projecting his own thoughts and feelings, such as his disappointment in his own wife or daughter, onto the patient ('counter-transference'). In the course of analysis, the patient is likely to display 'resistance' in the form of changing the topic, blanking out, falling asleep, arriving late, or missing appointments. Such behaviour is only to be expected, and indicates that the patient is close to recalling repressed material but afraid of doing so.

Aside from free association and dream interpretation, Freud recognized two further routes into the unconscious: parapraxes and jokes. Parapraxes, or slips of the tongue ('Freudian slips'), are essentially 'faulty actions' that occur when unconscious thoughts and desires suddenly parallel and then override conscious thoughts and intentions, for instance, calling a partner by the name of an ex-partner, substituting one word for another that rhymes or sounds similar ('I would like to thank/spank you'), or combining two words into a single one ('He is a very lustrous (illustrious/lustful) man'). Parapraxes often manifest in our speech, but can also manifest, among others, in our writing, misreadings, mishearings, and mislaying of objects and belongings. Freud reportedly 'joked' that 'there is no such thing as an accident'.

In *The Interpretation of Dreams*, Freud developed his 'topographical model' of the mind, describing the conscious, the unconscious, and an intermediary layer called the preconscious, which, although not conscious, could readily be accessed by the conscious. Freud later became dissatisfied with the topographical model and replaced it with the 'structural model', according to which the mind is split into the id, ego, and superego (Figure 5.3). The wholly unconscious id contains our drives and repressed emotions. The id is driven by the 'pleasure principle' and seeks out immediate gratification. But

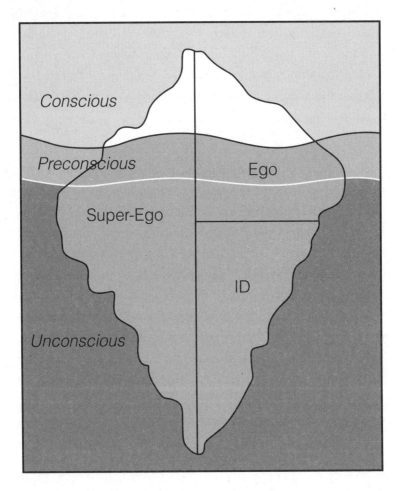

Figure 5.3. Freud's topographical (the ocean) and structural (the iceberg) models superimposed. Only the tip of the iceberg is conscious. In *The World as Will*, Schopenhauer, who anticipated Freud, compared the human intellect to a lame man who can see, riding on the shoulders of a blind giant.

in this it is opposed by the mostly unconscious superego, a sort of moral judge that arises from the internalization of parental figures, and, by extension, of society itself. Caught in the middle is the ego, which, in contrast to the id and superego, is mostly conscious. The function of the ego is to reconcile the id and the superego, and thereby to enable the person to engage successfully with reality.

For Freud, neurotic anxiety and other ego defences arise when the ego is overwhelmed by the demands of the id, the superego, and reality.

Although much derided in his time and still derided today, Freud is unquestionably one of the deepest and most original thinkers of the 20th century. Despite the disdain in which doctors often hold him, he is, ironically, the most famous of all doctors and the only one to have become a household name. He is credited with discovering the unconscious and inventing psychoanalysis, and had a colossal impact not only on his field of psychiatry but also on art, literature, and the humanities. He may have been thinking of himself (he often did) when he noted that, 'the voice of intelligence is soft, but it does not die until it has made itself heard.'

In his paper of 1943, *A Theory of Human Motivation*, psychologist Abraham Maslow proposed that healthy human beings had a certain number of needs, and that these needs are arranged in a hierarchy, with some needs (such as physiological and safety needs) being more primitive or basic than others (such as social and ego needs). Maslow's so-called 'hierarchy of needs' is often presented as a five-level pyramid, with higher needs coming into focus only once lower, more basic needs have been met (Figure 5.4).

Maslow called the bottom four levels of the pyramid 'deficiency needs' because we do not feel anything if they are met, but become anxious or distressed if they are not. Thus, physiological needs such as eating, drinking, and sleeping are deficiency needs, as are safety needs, social needs such as friendship and sexual intimacy, and ego needs such as self-esteem and recognition. On the other hand, he called the fifth, top level of the pyramid a 'growth need' because

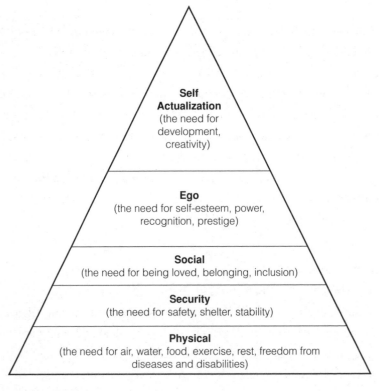

Figure 5.4. Maslow's hierarchy of needs.

our need to self-actualize enables us to fulfill our true and highest potential as human beings.

Once we have met our deficiency needs, the focus of our anxiety shifts to self-actualization, and we begin, even if only at a sub- or semi-conscious level, to contemplate our bigger picture. However, only a small minority of people is able to self-actualize because self-actualization requires uncommon qualities such as honesty, independence, awareness, objectivity, creativity, and originality.

Maslow's hierarchy of needs has been criticized for being overly schematic and lacking in scientific grounding, but it presents an intuitive and potentially useful theory of human motivation. After all, there is surely some truth in the popular saying that one cannot philosophize on an empty stomach, or in Aristotle's acute observation that, 'all paid work absorbs and degrades the mind'.

Many people who have met all their deficiency needs do not self-actualize, instead inventing more deficiency needs for themselves, because to contemplate the meaning of their life and of life in general would lead them to entertain the possibility of their meaninglessness and the prospect of their own death and annihilation.

A person who begins to contemplate his bigger picture may come to fear that life is meaningless and death inevitable, but at the same time cling on to the cherished belief that his life is eternal or important or at least significant. This gives rise to an inner conflict that is sometimes referred to as 'existential anxiety' or, more colourfully, 'the trauma of non-being'.

While fear and anxiety and their pathological forms are grounded in threats to life, existential anxiety is rooted in the brevity and apparent meaninglessness or absurdity of life. Existential anxiety is so disturbing and unsettling that most people avoid it at all costs, constructing a false reality out of goals, ambitions, habits, customs, values, culture, and religion so as to deceive themselves that their lives are special and meaningful and that death is distant or delusory.

However, such self-deception comes at a heavy price. According to Jean-Paul Sartre, people who refuse to face up to 'non-being' are acting in 'bad faith', and living out a life that is inauthentic and unfulfilling. Facing up to non-being can bring insecurity, loneliness, responsibility, and consequently anxiety, but it can also bring a sense of calm, freedom, and even nobility. Far from being pathological, existential anxiety is a sign of health, strength, and courage, and a harbinger of bigger and better things to come.

For theologian Paul Tillich (1886-1965), refusing to face up to non-being leads not only to a life that is inauthentic but also to pathological (or neurotic) anxiety.

In *The Courage to Be*, Tillich asserts:

> *He who does not succeed in taking his anxiety courageously upon himself can succeed in avoiding the extreme situation of despair by escaping into neurosis. He still affirms himself but on a limited scale. Neurosis is the way of avoiding nonbeing by avoiding being.*

According to this outlook, pathological anxiety, though seemingly grounded in threats to life, in fact arises from repressed existential anxiety, which itself arises from our uniquely human capacity for self-consciousness.

Facing up to non-being enables us to put our life into perspective, see it in its entirety, and thereby lend it a sense of direction and unity. If the ultimate source of anxiety is fear of the future, the future ends in death; and if the ultimate source of anxiety is uncertainty, death is the only certainty. It is only by facing up to death, accepting its inevitability, and integrating it into life that we can escape from the pettiness and paralysis of anxiety, and, in so doing, free ourselves to make the most out of our lives and out of ourselves.

Some philosophers have gone even further by asserting that the very purpose of life is none other than to prepare for death. In Plato's *Phaedo*, Socrates, who is not long to die, tells the philosophers Simmias and Cebes that absolute justice, absolute beauty, or absolute good cannot be apprehended with the eyes or any other bodily organ, but only by the mind or soul. Therefore, the philosopher seeks in as far as possible to separate body from soul and become pure soul. As death is the complete separation of body and soul, the philosopher aims at death, and indeed can be said to be almost dead.

Yet, the problem of hard meaning remains, and meaning is of crucial importance to our lives: a subjective lack of meaning is the most common reason for suicide in young and middle-aged people, and elderly people often suffer a precipitous decline in their mental and physical health if they are robbed of their sense of purpose. Many people go to great lengths to secure meaning through money, status, affiliations, and relationships. They may also attempt to extend their existence by having children and grandchildren, or else by leaving a significant artistic, intellectual, or social legacy.

But, as PB Shelley's *Ozymandias* makes chillingly clear, all this is merely to delay the inevitable:

> *'My name is Ozymandias, king of kings:*
> *Look on my works, ye Mighty, and despair!'*
> *Nothing beside remains. Round the decay*
> *Of that colossal wreck, boundless and bare*
> *The lone and level sands stretch far away.*

Some people are able to find meaning through religion or spirituality, but, for the first time in human history, many others are not. If we cannot find meaning through religion or spirituality, is it still possible for us to find some semblance of meaning?

First, we need to consider the possibility that life in general has no meaning, as this encourages us to see our life *sub specie aeternitatis* ('under the aspect of eternity') and so to put it into context and perspective. Second, we need to pursue valued goals and incentives that are outside ourselves such as devotion to humankind or philosophy. As such goals and incentives are universal, infinite, and to the benefit of others, they are likely to bring at least some measure of meaning. Third, our chosen goals and incentives need to bear a coherent relation to one another and form part of a unifying vision that can make them seem like more than a simple succession of isolated incidents. Such a unifying vision needs to be guided by carefully thought-through ideals, so that trying to meet it and live by it can be experienced as inspiring and motivating.

If these conditions can be met, the focus of attention shifts from the future to the present moment, and from the goal itself to the process of achieving that goal. Through immersion into the present, which is life, the future, which is death and anxiety, simply recedes into the background.

Chapter 6

Suicide and self-harm

And so it was I entered the broken world
To trace the visionary company of love, its voice
An instant in the wind (I know not whither hurled)
But not for long to hold each desperate choice.

—Hart Crane

S uicide is a neologism coined from *sui caedes*, Latin for 'murder of oneself', and has been defined by sociologist Emile Durkheim (1858-1917) as applying to 'all cases of death resulting directly or indirectly from a positive or negative act of the victim himself, which he knows will produce this result'.

Suicide can simply be defined as the act of intentionally killing oneself, although intentionally killing oneself with the primary aim of saving or helping others may be seen more as self-sacrifice than suicide. Thus, a revised and more restrictive definition of suicide might be, the act of intentionally killing oneself, *with the primary aim of dying.*

In some cases of suicide, the primary aim is not entirely clear. For example, in 1941 Virginia Woolf killed herself by walking into the River Ouse with a large rock in her pocket. In her suicide note to her husband, she attributes her suicide both to the deterioration in her mental illness and to her guilt at 'spoiling' her husband's life.

This is her heartrending suicide note:

> *Dearest, I feel certain I am going mad again. I feel we can't go through another of those terrible times. And I shan't recover this time. I begin to hear voices, and I can't concentrate. So I am doing what seems the best thing to do. You have given me the greatest possible happiness. You have been in every way all that anyone could be. I don't think two people could have been happier till this terrible disease came. I can't fight any longer. I know that I am spoiling your life, that without me you could work. And you will I know. You see I can't even write this properly. I can't read. What I want to say is I owe all the happiness of my life to you. You have been entirely patient with me and entirely good. I want to say that—everybody knows it. If anybody could have saved me it would have been you. Everything has gone from me but the certainty of your goodness. I can't go on spoiling your life any longer.*

> *I don't think two people could have been happier than we have been.*

> *V.*

Suicide should be distinguished from assisted suicide, the making available to a person of the information and/or means to end his life; and from voluntary euthanasia (Greek, 'good death'), the deliberate ending of the life of a person who has requested it. A more restrictive definition of euthanasia is, the deliberate ending of the life of an incurably ill person who has requested it, to relieve suffering. Active euthanasia, which in many jurisdictions is still looked upon as murder or manslaughter, involves the use of lethal substances or forces to kill, whereas passive euthanasia merely involves the withholding of common treatments such as antibiotics or surgery.

The act of suicide itself should be distinguished from other acts of self-harm, and particularly from attempted suicide and parasuicide (Figure 6.1). Attempted suicide is the act of trying to kill oneself (with intention), but failing to do so. Parasuicide is any act, or 'suicidal gesture', that resembles suicide but does not result in death. The intention of a parasuicidal act might have been to kill oneself, but it might also have been a means of attracting attention, a 'cry for help', an act of revenge, or an expression of despair, among others.

Suicide, attempted suicide, and parasuicide are all forms of (deliberate) self-harm, which can be defined as the act of intentionally injuring oneself, irrespective of the degree of injury sustained. Acts of self-harm such as self-cutting that are neither suicide, attempted suicide, nor parasuicide may be carried out for a variety

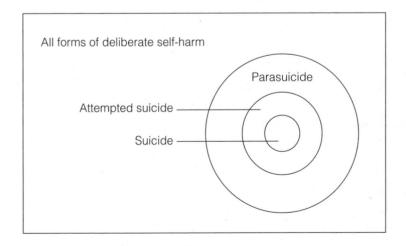

Figure 6.1. Venn diagram of the forms of deliberate self-harm.

of reasons, most commonly to express and relieve bottled-up anger or tension, feel more in control of a seemingly desperate life situation, or punish oneself for being a 'bad' person.

For some people, the pain inflicted by self-harm is preferable to the numbness and emptiness that it replaces: it is something rather than nothing, and a salutatory reminder that one is still able to feel, that one is still alive. For others, the pain of self-harm merely replaces a different kind of pain that they can neither understand nor control. Acts of self-harm reflect deep distress, and are most often used as a desperate and reluctant last resort—a means of surviving rather than dying, and sometimes also a means of attracting much-needed attention.

In general, it appears that teenagers, particularly teenage girls, are at the highest risk of self-harm. Perhaps this is because older people are more adept at dealing with their emotions; or because they are better at hiding their self-harming activity; or else because they self-harm only indirectly, for instance, by misusing alcohol or drugs.

Self-harm is reaching epidemic proportions in the UK. In a speech delivered to the Mental Health Conference in January 2015, the then Deputy Prime Minister Nick Clegg claimed that 'emergency departments see 300,000 cases of self-harm each year'. This in itself is a gross underestimate of the true incidence of self-harm, as the vast majority of cases never present to hospital.

According to the British Psychological Association and the Guardian, the most recent Health Behaviour in School-Aged Children (HBSC) report is due to reveal that, of 6,000 young people aged 11, 13, and 15 surveyed across England, about 20% of the 15-year-olds reported self-harming within the past 12 months.

The last similar survey of self-harm in England, published in the British Medical Journal in 2002, surveyed 6020 pupils aged 15 and 16. At the time, 'only' 6.9% of the pupils reported self-harming within the past 12 months, compared to about 20% in the 2013-14 HBSC study.

The vast majority of cases of self-harm that present to hospital involve either a tablet overdose or self-cutting, although self-cutting is much more common in the community at large. Occasionally, other forms of self-harm are also seen, such as banging or hitting body parts, scratching, hair pulling, burning, and strangulation. The drugs most commonly involved in tablet overdoses are painkillers, antidepressants, and sedatives.

According to the most recent report on self-harm in Oxford, England, of those people who present to hospital, about 25% report high suicidal intent, and about 40% are assessed as suffering from a 'major psychiatric disorder' excluding personality disorder and substance misuse. This suggests that many people who self-harm are not in fact mentally ill.

The problems most frequently cited at the time of presentation are problems with relationships, alcohol, employment or studies, finances, housing, social isolation, physical health, bereavement, and childhood emotional and sexual abuse.

For some people, self-harm is a one-off response to a severe emotional crisis. For others, it is a more long-term problem. People may keep on self-harming because they keep on suffering from the same problems, or they may stop self-harming for a time, sometimes several years, only to return to self-harm at the next major emotional crisis.

Self-harm is generally believed to be rare in many non-Western countries, suggesting that it is in fact a culture-bound syndrome (Chapter 5). Foreign doctors often claim never to have seen a case of self-harm prior to working in the UK.

The testimonial of Dr Eric Avevor in *The Psychiatrist* is fairly representative:

> *The subject [of self-harm] was hardly mentioned, let alone taught, as a topic throughout my undergraduate medical training in Ghana. In my medical school clinical years and throughout my work as a house officer in the largest teaching hospital in Ghana, I never saw or heard of a single case of self-harm. I later worked as a medical officer (hospital-based general practice) in a busy district hospital for three years and here too I never encountered such a case ... I had a cultural shock in my first psychiatric senior house officer post in the UK when I quickly realised that self-harm was the 'bread and butter' of emergency psychiatric practice.*

As Dr Avevor concedes, this stark difference could owe to under-reporting of cases in Ghana. But even if very common, under-reporting seems unlikely to account for the full difference.

In his speech to the Mental Health Conference, Nick Clegg said that, 'almost 4,700 people died by suicide in 2013 in England, just under 78% of whom were men, and suicide remains one of the biggest killers for men under the age of 50.' While self-harm may be more common in women, completed suicide is more than three times more common in men. This may be because men are more likely to use violent means of suicide, or because men with suicidal thoughts find it harder to obtain and engage with the help and support that they need.

According to the Office for National Statistics (ONS), the highest UK suicide rate in 2013 by broad age group was among men aged 45 to 59, at 25.1 deaths per 100,000—the highest for that age group since 1981.

An important problem with figures such as these is that they reflect reported suicides, which in turn reflect verdicts reached by coroners' inquests. *Actual* suicide rates may be considerably higher than the statistics suggest, particularly in elderly people in whom suicide is more likely to be mistaken for a natural death.

The WHO estimates that, each year, there are about 800,000 deaths by suicide in the world, which equates to an annual global suicide rate of 11.4 per 100,000 people. Globally, suicide accounts for 1.4% of deaths, making it the 15th leading cause of death overall and the leading cause of death among 15-29 year olds. Rates of attempted suicide are, of course, much higher still.

As methods of reporting suicide vary from one country to another, it is difficult to make robust international comparisons. However, it seems that, in high-income countries, middle-aged men have the highest suicide rates, whereas in low- and middle-income countries it is young adults and elderly women.

In Europe, there is a tendency for suicide rates to increase the more north and the more east one travels. According to the WHO, in 2012, suicide rates in Russia, Lithuania, and Latvia exceeded 30 per 100,000. This compared to 6.3 per 100,000 in Greece, 7.6 in Italy, 8.2 in Spain, 9.8 in the UK, and 19.4 in the US.

Several factors can affect the suicide rate, including the time of year, the state of the economy, and media headlines.

Contrary to popular belief, the suicide rate peaks in the springtime, not the wintertime. This may be because the rebirth that marks springtime accentuates feelings of hopelessness in those already prone to suicide, or because people who are depressed cannot muster the energy to carry through with suicide in the winter.

It comes as no surprise that the suicide rate increases during times of economic depression. More unexpected, however, is that it also increases during times of economic prosperity, presumably because people feel 'left behind' if every Tom, Dick, and Harry seems to be racing ahead. Although economists focus on the absolute size of salaries, several sociological studies have found that the effect of money on happiness results less from the things that money can buy (absolute income effect) than from comparing one's income to that of others, and particularly to that of one's peers (relative income effect). This could help explain the finding that people in developed countries such as the US and UK are no happier than 50 or 60 years ago. Despite being considerably richer, healthier, and more leisured, they have only barely managed to 'keep up with the Joneses'.

On the other hand, the suicide rate decreases during times of national cohesion or coming together, such as during a war or its modern substitute, the international sporting event. During such times, there is a feeling of 'being in it together' along with a mix of curiosity, suspense, and anticipation. For example, a study looking at England and Wales found that the number of suicides reported for the month of September 2001 was significantly lower than for any other month of that year, and lower than for any month of September in 22 years. According to the author of the study, these findings 'support Durkheim's theory that periods of external threat create group integration within society and lower the suicide rate through the impact of social cohesion'.

Like so much else, suicidal behaviour is culturally shaped. Thus, the suicide rate rises after the depiction or prominent reporting of a suicide in the media. A suicide that is inspired by another suicide, either in the media or in real life, is sometimes referred to as a 'copycat suicide', and the phenomenon itself as the 'Werther effect'. In 1774, polymath JW Goethe (1749-1832) published a novel entitled *The Sorrows of Young Werther*, in which the fictional Werther shoots himself following an ill-fated romance. Within no time, young men from all over Europe began committing suicide using exactly the same method as Werther, prompting the novel to be banned in several places. In some cases, suicide can spread through an entire local community with one copycat suicide inspiring the next. Such a 'suicide contagion' is most likely to occur in impressionable and vulnerable population groups such as disaffected teenagers.

At the individual level, a person's risk of committing suicide can be increased by a number of demographic and social risk factors. Demographic risk factors for suicide, at least in the West, include being male; being relatively young; and being single, widowed, separated, or divorced. Social risk factors for suicide include having recently suffered a life crisis such as losing a close friend or relative; being unemployed, insecurely employed, or retired; and having a poor level of social support as is often the case for the elderly, prisoners, immigrants, refugees, and the bereaved. Certain occupational groups such as veterinary surgeons, farmers, pharmacists, and doctors have been found to be at a higher risk of suicide. This probably owes to their training and skills, and to their privileged access to highly lethal means such as prescription-only drugs and firearms.

As well as demographic and social risk factors, a person's risk of committing suicide can be increased by a number of clinical risk factors. Indeed, the most important predictor of suicide is a previous episode of self-harm, and a person's risk of completing suicide in the year following an episode of self-harm is approximately 100 times greater than the average. Conversely, up to half of all people who complete suicide have a history of self-harm.

Suicidal behaviour tends to cluster in families, so a family history of suicide or self-harm also increases suicide risk. Perhaps this is because suicide is a learnt behaviour, or, more likely, because family members share a genetic predisposition to mental disorders such as schizophrenia and bipolar disorder that are associated with a higher risk of suicide.

Also at a higher risk of suicide are people with a mental disorder who are not responding to, or complying with, their prescribed medication; and people experiencing certain psychotic symptoms such as delusions of persecution, delusions of control, delusions of jealousy, delusions of guilt, second person command hallucinations (for example, a voice saying, 'Take that knife and kill yourself'), and passivity, which is the sense that one's thoughts, feelings, or actions are being controlled by an external agency.

Physical illnesses also increase suicide risk. This is particularly true of physical illnesses that are terminal, that involve long-term pain or disability, or that affect the brain. Physical illnesses that have been associated with an increased suicide rate include cancer, coronary heart disease, chronic obstructive pulmonary disease, early-onset diabetes, stroke, epilepsy, multiple sclerosis, and AIDS.

According to the ONS, the most common method of suicide in the UK in 2013 was 'hanging, strangulation and suffocation', which accounted for 56.1% of male and 40.2% of female suicides. This is astonishingly high in so far as hanging is both violent and ineffectual, and serves to highlight the important influence of culture and tradition on chosen methods of suicide.

For the first time in 2013, 'hanging, strangulation and suffocation' overtook poisoning as the most common method of suicide in women. In 2013, poisoning accounted for 38% of female suicides, down from 49% in 2002. Drowning, falls, and other methods remained fairly constant over the period.

Methods of suicide are influenced not only by culture but also by availability and accessibility. Thus, the proliferation of barbiturates in the early 1960s led to a marked increase in poisoning as a method of suicide, and gunshot as a method of suicide is far more common in the US than it is in the UK. A small proportion of suicides involve a suicide pact in which two or more people—usually an elderly couple rather than a pair of star-cross'd lovers—agree to commit suicide at or around the same time.

The Roman Catholic Church has long argued that one's life is the property of God and thus that to commit suicide is to deride God's prerogatives. The counterargument, by philosopher David Hume (1711-1776) is that, if such is the case, then to save someone's life is also to deride God's prerogatives.

Most religions share the Church's belief in the sanctity of life, although a few have come to regard at least some suicides as honourable. For example, a number of Tibetan monks have killed themselves in protest against the Chinese occupation of Tibet—although this is perhaps more a case of self-sacrifice than suicide proper.

Legal systems have historically been informed by religion, such that in many jurisdictions suicide and attempted suicide are still illegal. The very expression 'commit suicide' implies or at least suggests a crime or sin. In late 2014, the Indian government moved to decriminalize 'attempt to suicide' by deleting Section 209 of the Penal Code from the statute book. Under the said section, a suicide bid could be punished with a prison term of up to one year.

In the UK, the Suicide Act of 1961 decriminalized attempted suicide and suicide, but voluntary euthanasia remains a crime. This may change as the voice of pro-choicers becomes louder than that of pro-lifers. Broadly speaking, pro-choicers argue that a person's life belongs to no one but himself, and that his decision to commit suicide, especially if justified as a rational solution to real problems such as chronic and disabling pain, should be respected and assisted. In contrast, pro-lifers believe that a person's life is not his to take, regardless of circumstances.

Some of the stronger arguments in favour of voluntary euthanasia are that it preserves dignity, prevents suffering, and frees up valuable healthcare resources. On the other side of the argument, a person with a physical or mental disorder may lack the mental capacity to make a rational decision about such an important issue, or may feel pressured into making a decision, and, of course, cannot change his mind once he is dead. Moreover, voluntary euthanasia is difficult to regulate, and could be open to abuse by doctors and relatives keen to unburden themselves and free up or inherit resources.

Unlike most people, some philosophers do not think about suicide in terms of ethics. Existentialist philosophers in particular turn the tables round by arguing that life has no meaning and therefore that there is no reason *not* to commit suicide. Rather, a person must justify not committing suicide by giving his life a meaning and fulfilling his unique potential through this meaning.

As Jean-Paul Sartre mused:

> *One is still what one is going to cease to be and already what one is going to become. One lives one's death, one dies one's life.*

Nihilistic (from the Latin *nihil*, 'nothing') philosophers differ from existentialist philosophers in that they believe that a person cannot justify his life even by giving it an individual meaning. For nihilistic philosophers, nothing can have a meaning, not even suicide itself.

Interesting as this may all be, suicide is seldom the product of rational deliberation, the so-called 'rational suicide', but mostly an act of uncontrollable anguish and despair.

Around 1755, David Hume, who suffered from melancholy, published *On Suicide* and *On the Immortality of the Soul* in a book of essays entitled *Five Dissertations*. Unfortunately, pre-release copies of *Five Dissertations* stirred up such controversy that both essays had to be removed.

In *On Suicide*, Hume argues that, though only 'one step' could put an end to his misery, man dares not commit suicide because of 'a vain fear lest he offend his Maker'. This, combined with his natural fear of death, makes it 'all the more difficult for him to be free'. Hume proposes to 'restore men to their native liberty' by examining all the common arguments against suicide and demonstrating that suicide is 'free from every imputation of guilt or blame'.

According to Hume, God established the laws of nature and enabled all animals, including man, to make use of them by entrusting them with certain bodily and mental powers. Owing to this interaction between the laws of nature and the powers of animals, God has no need to be involved in the world: '...the providence of the Deity appears not immediately in any operation, but governs everything by those general and immutable laws, which have been established from the beginning of time.'

Given this state of affairs, man employs the powers with which he has been invested to provide as best as possible for his 'ease, happiness, or preservation'. If this should bring him to commit suicide, then so be it: the interaction between the laws of nature and the powers of man clearly permit it, so why should it pose an exception? Thus, suicide is permissible even if one adopts a religious stance.

For Hume:

> *The life of man is of no greater importance to the universe than that of an oyster... I thank Providence, both for the good which I have already enjoyed, and for the power with which I am endowed of escaping the ill that threatens me.*

Natural philosopher Pliny the Elder (23-79) goes one step further than Hume in his *Natural History* by regarding the ability to commit suicide as the one advantage that man possesses over God:

> *God cannot give himself death even if he wishes, but man can do so at any time he chooses.*

A common argument against suicide is that it is selfish and harms the individuals and society that are left behind. For Hume, a person does no harm in committing suicide, but merely ceases to do good. Assuming that he is under some obligation to do good, this obligation comes to an end with death; and even if it does not, and he is under a perpetual obligation to do good, this should not come at the expense of greater harm to himself, that is, at the expense of prolonging a miserable existence for some 'frivolous advantage that the public may perhaps receive'. In some cases, a person may have become a burden to society, and so may actually do most good by committing suicide. In such cases, says Hume, suicide is better than morally neutral. It is morally good.

Regardless of the morality or permissibility of committing suicide, suicide entails death, and so the question naturally arises as to whether death should or should not be feared. In his influential paper of 1970, tersely entitled *Death*, philosopher Thomas Nagel (born 1937) addresses precisely this question: if death is the permanent end of our existence, is it an evil?

Either death is an evil because it deprives us of life, or it is a mere blank because there is no one left to experience this deprivation. Thus, if death is an evil, this is not in virtue of any positive attribute that it has, but in virtue of what it deprives us from, namely, life. For Nagel, the bare experience of life is intrinsically valuable, regardless of the balance of its good and bad elements.

The longer we are alive, the more we 'accumulate' life. In contrast, death cannot be accumulated—it is not 'an evil of which Shakespeare has so far received a larger portion than Proust'. Most people would not consider the temporary suspension of life as an evil, nor would they regard the long period before they were born as an evil. Therefore, if death is an evil this is not because it involves a period of non-existence, but because it deprives us of life.

Nagel draws three objections to this view, but only so as to later counter them. First, it is doubtful whether anything can be an evil unless it actually causes displeasure. Second, in the case of death there is no subject left on whom to impute an evil. As long as we exist, we have not yet died; and once we have died, we no longer exist. So there seems to be no time at which the evil of death might occur. Third, if most people would not regard the long period before they were born as an evil, then why should they regard the period after they are dead any differently?

Nagel counters these three objections by arguing that the good or evil that befalls us depends on our history and possibilities rather than on our momentary state, such that an evil can befall us even if we are not here to experience it. For instance, if an intelligent person receives a head injury that reduces his mental condition to that of a contented infant, this should be considered a serious evil even if the person himself (in his current state) is oblivious to his fate.

Thus, if the three objections are invalid, it is essentially because they ignore the direction of time.

Even though we cannot survive our death, we can still suffer evil; and even though we do not exist during the time before our birth and the time after our death, the time after our death is time of which we have been deprived, time in which we could have carried on enjoying the good of living.

The question remains as to whether the non-realization of further life is an absolute evil, or whether this depends on what can naturally be hoped for: the death of Keats at 24 is commonly regarded as tragic, but that of Tolstoy at 82 (even though he died of pneumonia in a hitherto obscure train station) is not.

'The trouble,' says Nagel, 'is that life familiarizes us with the goods of which death deprives us... Death, no matter how inevitable, is an abrupt cancellation of indefinitely extensive goods.'

Epilogue

'Mental disorder' is difficult to define. Generally speaking, mental disorders are conditions that involve either loss of contact with reality or distress and impairment. These experiences lie on a continuum of normal human experience, and so it is impossible to define the precise point at which they become pathological. Furthermore, concepts such as borderline personality disorder, schizophrenia, and depression listed in classifications of mental disorders may not map onto any real or distinct disease entities; even if they do, the symptoms and clinical manifestations that define them are open to subjective interpretation.

In an attempt to address these problems, classifications of mental disorders adopt a 'menu of symptoms' approach, and rigidly define each symptom in technical terms that are often far removed from a person's felt experience. This encourages health professionals to focus too closely on validating and treating an abstract diagnosis, and not enough on the person's distress, its context, and its significance or meaning.

Despite using complex aetiological models, health professionals tend to overlook that a person's felt experience often has a meaning in and of itself, even if it is broad, complex, or hard to fathom. By being helped to discover this meaning, the person may be able to identify and address the source of his distress, and so to make a faster, more complete, and more durable recovery. Beyond even this, he may gain important insights into himself, and a more refined and nuanced perspective over his life and life in general. These are rare and precious opportunities, and not to be squandered.

A more fundamental problem with labelling human distress and deviance as mental disorder is that it reduces a complex, important, and distinct part of human life to nothing more than a biological illness or defect, not to be processed or understood, or in some cases even embraced, but to be 'treated' and 'cured' by any means possible—often with drugs that may be doing much more harm than good. This biological reductiveness, along with the stigma that it attracts, shapes the person's interpretation and experience of his distress or deviance, and, ultimately, his relation to himself, to others, and to the world.

Moreover, to call out every difference and deviance as mental disorder is also to circumscribe normality and define sanity, not as tranquillity or possibility, which are the products of the wisdom that is being denied, but as conformity, placidity, and a kind of mediocrity.

Other pressing problems with the current medical model is that it encourages false epidemics, most glaringly in bipolar disorder and ADHD, and the wholesale exportation of Western mental disorders and Western accounts of mental disorder. Taken together, this is leading to a pandemic of Western disease categories and treatments, while undermining the variety and richness of the human experience.

Many critics question the scientific evidence underpinning such a robust biological approach and call for a radical rethink of mental disorders, not as detached disease processes that can be cut up into diagnostic labels, but as subjective and meaningful experiences grounded in personal and larger sociocultural narratives.

Unlike 'mere' medical or physical disorders, mental disorders are not just problems. If successfully navigated, they can also present opportunities. Simply acknowledging this can empower people to heal themselves and, much more than that, to grow from their experiences.

At the same time, mental disorders should not be romanticized or left unattended simply because they may or may not predispose to problem solving, personal development, or creativity. Some mental disorders undeniably have a strong biological basis, and all mental disorders are drab and intensely painful. In some cases, mental disorder can lead to serious harm and even to death by accident, self-neglect, or self-harm.

Rather than being medicalized or romanticized, mental disorders, or mental dis-eases, should be understood as nothing less or more than what they are, an expression of our deepest human nature. By recognizing their traits in ourselves and reflecting upon them, we may be able both to contain them and to put them to good use.

This is, no doubt, the highest form of genius.

The most beautiful things are those that are whispered by madness and written down by reason. We must steer a course between the two, close to madness in our dreams, but close to reason in our writing.

—André Gide

Notes

Epigraph

1. Nietzsche F (1883): *Thus Spake Zarathustra: A Book For All and None*, Pt. 1, Ch. 7 'On Reading and Writing'.

Introduction

2. Department of Health (2011): *No Health Without Mental Health: A Cross-Government Mental Health Outcomes Strategy for People of All Ages.*

3. Wittchen H-U and Jacobi F (2005): Size and burden of mental disorders in Europe—a critical review and appraisal of 27 studies. *European Neuropsychopharmacology* 15(4): 357-76.

4. Kessler RC et al. (2005): Lifetime prevalence and age-of-onset distributions of DSM-IV disorders in the National Comorbidity Survey Replication. *Archives of General Psychiatry* 62(6): 593-602.

5. National Health Interview Survey data 1997-2012.

6. Spence R et al. (2014): *Focus On: Antidepressant prescribing.* QualityWatch report from the Health Foundation and the Nuffield Trust.

7. Turner EH et al. (2008): Selective publication of antidepressant trials and its influence on apparent efficacy. *New England Journal of Medicine* 358(3):252-60.

8. Kirsch I et al. (2008): Initial Severity and Antidepressant Benefits: A Meta-Analysis of Data Submitted to the Food and Drug Administration. *PLoS Medicine* 5(2):e45.

9.   Isaac M et al. (2007): Schizophrenia outcome measures in the wider international community. *British Journal of Psychiatry* 191 (suppl. 50), s71-s77.

10.   Carroll L (1865): *Alice's Adventures in Wonderland*, Ch. 6.

1: Personality and personality disorders

11.   *Bible*, OT, Genesis 3:19 (KJV).

12.   Harlow JM (1868): Recovery from the passage of an iron bar through the head. *Publications of the Massachusetts Medical Society* 2:327-347.

13.   Harlow JM (1848): Passage of an iron rod through the head. *Boston Medical and Surgical Journal* 39:389-393.

14.   Jung CG (1934): The Development of Personality. *Collected Works*, 17, para. 289.

15.   Kierkegaard S (1846): *Concluding Unscientific Postscript to the Philosophical Fragments*.

16.   Sartre J-P (1944): *Huis Clos (No Exit)*, Act 1, Sc. 5. ...*l'enfer, c'est les autres*.

17.   Locke J (1689): *An Essay Concerning Human Understanding*, Ch. 27 'Of Identity and Diversity'.

18.   Shoemaker S (1963): *Self-knowledge and Self-identity*. Cornell University Press.

19.   Frankfurt HG (1969): Alternative possibilities and moral responsibility. *Journal of Philosophy* 66: 829-839.

20.   Strawson G (1986): *Freedom and Belief*. Oxford University Press.

21.   Theophrastus: *The Characters*.

22.   Pinel P (1801): *Traité medico-philosophique sur l'aliénation mentale; ou la manie (A Treatise on Insanity)*.

23.   Prichard JC (1835): *Treatise on Insanity and Other Disorders Affecting the Mind*.

24. Kraepelin E (1883): *Compendium der Psychiatrie*.

25. Schneider K (1923): *Die psychopathischen Persönlichkeiten* (*Psychopathic Personalities*).

26. American Psychiatric Association (2013): *Diagnostic and Statistical Manual of Mental Disorders, Fifth Edition*.

27. Kendler KS et al. (2006): Dimensional representations of DSM-IV cluster A personality disorders in a population-based sample of Norweigian twins: a multivariate study. *Psychological Medicine* 36(11):1583-91.

28. Macdonald JM (1963): The threat to kill. *American Journal of Psychiatry* 120: 125-130.

29. Kiehl KA & Buckholtz JW (2010): Inside the mind of a psychopath. *Scientific American Mind*, September/October 22-29.

30. Ovid: *Metamorphoses*, Bk. 3.

31. Lenzenweger MF (2008): Epidemiology of Personality Disorders. *Psychiatric Clinics of North America* 31(3):395-403.

32. Board BJ and Fritzon KF (2005): Disordered personalities at work. *Psychology, Crime and Law* 11:17-23.

33. James W (1902): *The Varieties of Religious Experience*, Lecture 1 'Religion and Neurology', Footnote 6.

34. Mullins-Sweat S et al. (2010): The Search for the Successful Psychopath. *Journal of Research in Personality* 44:554-558.

35. Hare RD (1998): *Without Conscience: The disturbing world of the psychopaths among us*, opening lines. Guilford Press.

36. Eisenstadt JM (1978): Parental loss and genius. *American Psychologist* 33:211-223.

37. Brown F (1968): Bereavement and lack of a parent in childhood. In: Miller E, *Foundations of Child Psychiatry*. Pergamon.

38. Aristotle: *Nicomachean Ethics*, Bk. 2.

39. Aristotle: *Nicomachean Ethics*, Bk. 10.

40. Wittgenstein L (1928): *Culture and Value*.

41. Gibbon E (1788): *The Decline and Fall of the Roman Empire*, Vol. 5, Ch. 50.

42. *Bhagavad Gita*, Ch. 18, 20-22.

43. *Bhagavad Gita*, Ch. 2, 12-13.

2: Schizophrenia, the price for being human

44. Szasz T (1973): *The Second Sin*. Doubleday.

45. Eugen Bleuler first introduced the term 'schizophrenia' in a lecture in Berlin on April 24, 1908, and then more formally in his seminal study of 1911, *Dementia Praecox, or the Group of Schizophrenias*.

46. Stevenson, RL (1886): *Strange Case of Dr Jekyll and Mr Hyde*.

47. Kraepelin E (1893): *Lehrbuch der Psychiatrie*.

48. *Bible*, OT, Samuel 16:14, 23 (KJV).

49. Euripides: *Herakles*.

50. Homer: *Iliad*, Bk. 19.

51. Hippocrates: *The Holy Disease*.

52. Cicero: *Tusculan Disputations*, Bk. 3 'On Grief of Mind'.

53. Weyer J (1563): *De Praestigiis Daemonum et Incantationibus ac Venificiis* (*On the Illusions of the Demons and on Spells and Poisons*, or *On the Deception of Demons*).

54. e.g. Locke J (1689): *An Essay Concerning Human Understanding*.

55. Pinel P (1801): *Traité medico-philosophique sur l'aliénation mentale; ou la manie* (*A Treatise on Insanity*).

56. Esquirol JE (1838): *Des maladies mentales considérées sous les rapports médical, hygiénique et medico-légal* (*Concerning Mental Illnesses*).

57. Kraepelin E (1883): *Compendium der Psychiatrie*.

58. Kraepelin E (1899): *Compendium der Psychiatrie*, 6th Ed.

59. Jaspers K (1913): *Allgemeine Psychopathologie* (*General Psychopathology*).

60. Brown BS (1976): The Life of Psychiatry. *American Journal of Psychiatry* 133:489-495. *From 1945 to 1955, it was nearly impossible for a non-psychoanalyst to become a chairman of a department or professor of psychiatry.*

61. Moncrieff J (2009): *The Myth of the Chemical Cure: A Critique of Psychiatric Drug Treatment*. Palgrave Macmillan.

62. Harrow M et al. (2012): Do all schizophrenia patients need antipsychotic treatment continuously throughout their lifetime? A 20-year longitudinal study. *Psychological Medicine* 42(10):2145-55.

63. For example, Crow TJ (1997): Schizophrenia as failure of hemispheric dominance for language. *Trends in Neuroscience* 20(8):339-43.

64. Crow TJ (1997): Is Schizophrenia the price that Homo sapiens pays for language? *Schizophrenia Research* 28:127-141. *Schizophrenia is not just an illness of humans, it may be THE illness of humanity.*

65. *Bible*, NT, John 1:1 (KJV).

66. Kyaga S et al. (2011): Creativity and mental disorder: family study of 300,000 people with severe mental disorder. *British Journal of Psychiatry* 199:373-379.

67. Folley BS & Park S (2005): Verbal creativity and schizotypal personality in relation to prefrontal hemispheric laterality: a behavioural and near-infrared optical imaging study. *Schizophrenia Research* 80(2-3):271-82.

68. Nettle D & Clegg H (2005): Schizotypy, creativity, and mating success in humans. *Proceedings of the Royal Society*, B 273:611-15.

69. Ohayon MM (2000): Prevalence of hallucinations and their pathological associations in the general population. *Psychiatry Research* 97(2-3):153-64.

70. Pirsig R (2006): Zen and the art of Robert Pirsig. Interview by Tim Adams in the November 19 issue of *The Observer*.

71. Plato (1973): *Phaedrus and the Seventh and Eighth Letters*. Trans. Walter Hamilton. Penguin.

72. Seneca the Younger: *De Tranquillitate Animi* (*On the Tranquillity of the Mind*), 17. *Nullum magnum ingenium sine mixture dementiae fuit.*

73. Cicero: *Tusculan Disputations* I. 33. 80; also in *On Divination* I. 37.

74. Shakespeare (c.1590): *A Midsummer Night's Dream*, Act V, Sc. 1.

75. Dryden J (1681): *Absalom and Achitophel*, Pt. 1, lines 163-164.

76. Pizzagalli D (2000): Brain electric correlates of strong belief in paranormal phenomena: intracerebral EEG source and regional Omega complexity analyses. *Psychiatry Research* 100(3):139-54.

77. Bonnie R (2002): Political Abuse of Psychiatry in the Soviet Union and China: Complexities and Controversies. *Journal of American Academic Psychiatry and the Law* 30:136-44.

78. U.S. Department of State Bureau of Democracy, Human Rights, and Labor: *Country Reports on Human Rights Practices for 2014: China (includes Tibet, Hong Kong, and Macau)*.

79. Rajneesh/Osho (1975): *The Mustard Seed: Discourses on the sayings of Jesus taken from the Gospel according to Thomas*, Ch. 9. Rajneesh Foundation.

80. Rosenhan D (1973): On being sane in insane places. *Science* 179:250-258.

81. Szasz TS (1961): *The Myth of Mental Illness: Foundations of a Theory of Personal Conduct*. Harper Perennial, 2010.

82. Szasz TS (1976): Schizophrenia: the sacred symbol of psychiatry. *British Journal of Psychiatry* 129:308-16.

83. Foucault, M (1961): *Folie et Déraison: Histoire de la folie à l'âge classique* (*Madness and Civilization: A History of Insanity in the Age of Reason/History of Madness*). Plon.

84. For example, Laing RD (1960): *The Divided Self: An Existential Study in Sanity and Madness*. Penguin.

85. Jung CG (1960): Psychogenesis of Mental Disease 362, in *Collected Works of C.G. Jung*, Vol. 3. Princeton University Press.

3: Depression, the curse of the strong

86. *Bible*, OT, Ecclesiastes 1:17-18 (KJV).

87. Styron W (1990): *Darkness Visible: A Memoir of Madness*. Vintage Classic 2001.

88. Daniel Pagnin et al. (2004): Efficacy of ECT in Depression: A Meta-Analytic Review. *Journal of ECT* 20:13-20.

89. UK ECT Review Group (2003): Efficacy and safety of electroconvulsive therapy in depressive disorders: a systematic review and meta-analysis. *Lancet* 361:799-808.

90. Read J & Bentall R (2010): The effectiveness of electroconvulsive therapy: A literature review. *Epidemiologica e Psychiatria Sociale* 19:333-347.

91. Turner EH et al. (2008): Selective publication of antidepressant trials and its influence on apparent efficacy. *New England Journal of Medicine* 358(3):252-60.

92. Kirsch I et al. (2008): Initial Severity and Antidepressant Benefits: A Meta-Analysis of Data Submitted to the Food and Drug Administration. *PLoS Medicine* 5(2):e45.

93. Watson JB & Rayner R (1920): Conditioned emotional reaction. *Journal of Experimental Psychology* 3:1-14.

94. Benedetti F et al. (2011): How Placebos Change the Patient's Brain. *Neuropsychopharmacology* 36(1):339-354.

95. Burgess A (1962): *A Clockwork Orange*. William Heinemann.

96. Voting numbers at the 1973 APA convention are from Davies J (2013): *Cracked: Why Psychiatry is Doing More Harm Than Good*. Icon Books.

97. *Talmud*, Kiddushin 36.

98. Thorndike EL (1928): *The Fundamentals of Learning*. Teachers College Press.

99. Skinner BF (1969): *Contingencies of Reinforcement: A Theoretical Analysis*. Meredith.

100. Watson JB (1930): *Behaviorism* (Revised edition). University of Chicago Press.

101. Cuijpers P et al. (2008): Psychotherapy for depression in adults: A meta-analysis of comparative outcome studies. *Journal of Consulting and Clinical Psychology* 76(6):909-922.

102. Johnsen TJ & Friborg O (2015): The effects of cognitive behavioral therapy as an anti-depressive treatment is falling: A meta-analysis. *Psychological Bulletin* 141(4):747-68.

103. 101. Frankl VE (1946): *Man's Search for Meaning: An Introduction to Logotherapy*. Beacon Press. Trans. Ilse Lasch.

104. *Bible*, OT, Psalms 41:8.

105. Keedwell P (2008): *How Sadness Survived: The Evolutionary Basis of Depression*. Radcliffe Publishing.

106. Proust M (1927): *In Search of Lost Time: The Past Recaptured*.

107. Dante (1320): *The Divine Comedy: Hell*, opening verses. Trans. Neel Burton.

4: Bipolar disorder, that fine madness

108. Plato, *Phaedrus*. Trans. Walter Hamilton.

109. Udachina A & Mansell W (2007): Cross-validation of the Mood Disorders Questionnaire, the Internal State Scale, and the Hypomanic Personality Scale. *Personality and Individual Differences* 42(8):1539-1549.

110. Allen Frances in conversation with James Davis, as quoted in Davies J (2013): *Cracked: Why Psychiatry is Doing More Harm Than Good*. Icon Books.

111. National Health Interview Survey data 1997-2012.

112. Kirkey S (2015): Speed-like stimulants prescribed for adult ADHD part of 'psychiatric fad,' risk being used for mental edge. *The National Post*, July 23, 2015.

113. Cosgrove L & Drimsky L (2012): A comparison of DSM-IV and DSM-5 panel members' financial associations with industry: A pernicious problem persists. *PLOS Medicine* 9(3):e1001190.

114. Ruskin, J (1833), as quoted in a letter to his father dated 15 January.

115. As quoted in, Sims A (1988): *Symptoms in the Mind: An Introduction to Descriptive Psychopathology*. Ballière Tindal.

116. Kerner B (2014): Genetics of Bipolar Disorder. *Journal of the Application of Clinical Genetics* 7:33-42. '…about half of the individuals with bipolar disorder attempt suicide at least once in their lifetime, and many complete the attempt.'

117. Crump C. et al. (2013): Comorbidities and Mortality in Bipolar Disorder: A Swedish National Cohort Study. *JAMA Psychiatry* 70(9):931-939.

118. Simpson SG & Jamison KR (1999): The risk of suicide in patients with bipolar disorders. *Journal of Clinical Psychiatry* 60 Suppl 2:53-6.

119. Aretaeus of Cappadocia: *Causes and Symptoms of Chronic Diseases*, Bk. 1, Ch. 6 'On Madness'.

120. Jamison KR (1996): *Touched with Fire: Manic-Depressive Illness and the Artistic Temperament*. Simon and Schuster.

121. Poe EA (1850): *Eleanora*.

122. Woolf V (1925): *Mrs Dalloway*.

123. Woolf V (1930): Letter to Ethel Smyth dated Sunday, 22nd June.

124. Andreasen NC (1987): Creativity and mental illness: Prevalence rates in writers and their first-degree relatives. *American Journal of Psychiatry* 144:1288-1292.

125. Jamison K (1989): Mood disorders and patterns of creativity in British authors and artists. *Psychiatry* 52:125-34.

126. Tsuchiya KJ et al. (2004): Higher socio-economic status of parents may increase risk for bipolar disorder in the offspring. *Psychological Medicine* 34(5):787-93.

127. Smoller JW & Finn CT (2003): Family, twin, and adoption studies of bipolar disorder. *American Journal of Medical Genetics* 123C(1):48-58.

128. Lichtenstein P et al. (2009): Common genetic determinants of schizophrenia and bipolar disorder in Swedish families: a population-based study. *Lancet* 373(9659):234-239.

129. Nietzsche F (1883): *Thus Spoke Zarathustra*, First Part, Zarathustra's Prologue.

130. Jauk E (2013): The relationship between intelligence and creativity: New support for the threshold hypothesis by means of empirical breakpoint detection. *Intelligence* 41(4):212-221.

131. Tchaikovsky P. (1878). Letter to Frau von Meck, dated March 17th, 1878, in: *The Life and Letters of Peter Ilich Tchaikovsky*. Ed. & trans. R. Newmarch (1905).

132. Plato: *Ion*. Trans. Benjamin Jowett.

133. Post, F. (1994): Creativity and psychopathology. A study of 291 world-famous men. *British Journal of Psychiatry* 165(1):22-34.

134. Storr A (1988): *Solitude*, p143. Flamingo.

135. Santosa CM et al. (2007): Enhanced creativity in bipolar disorder patients: a controlled study. *Journal of Affective Disorders* 100(1-3):31-9.

136. Santosa CM et al. (2007): Temperament-creativity relationships in mood disorder patients, healthy controls and highly creative individuals. *Journal of Affective Disorders* 100(1-3):41-8.

137. Tremblay CH et al. (2010): Brainstorm: occupational choice, bipolar illness and creativity. *Economics & Human Biology* 8(2):233-41.

138. Andreasen N (2008): The relationship between creativity and mood disorders. *Dialogues in Clinical Neuroscience* 10(2):251-255.

139. Rilke RM (1912), in a letter to Emil Freiherr von Gebsattel dated 24 January 1912. *So viel, wie ich mich kenne, scheint mir sicher, daß, wenn man mir meine Teufel austriebe, auch meinem Engeln ein kleiner, ein ganz kleiner (sagen wir) Shrecken geschähe, … und gerade darauf darf ich es auf keinen Preis ankommen lassen.*

140. Moncrieff J (2015): *Reasons not to believe in lithium.* Posted on July 1, 2015 on joannamoncrieff.com. http://joannamoncrieff.com/2015/07/01/reasons-not-to-believe-in-lithium/

141. Jamison KR (1996): *An Unquiet Mind: A Memoir of Moods and Madness.* Vintage.

5: *Anxiety, freedom, and death*

142. Kierkegaard S (1844): *The Concept of Anxiety: A Simple Psychologically Orienting Deliberation on the Dogmatic Issue of Hereditary Sin*, p61. Trans. Reidar Thomte. Princeton University Press 1980.

143. Kessler RC et al (2005): Prevalence, severity, and comorbidity of twelve-month DSM-IV disorders in the National Comorbidity Survey Replication (NCS-R). *Archives of General Psychiatry* 62(6):617-27.

144. For example, Jacob RG et al. (1996): Panic, agoraphobia, and vestibular dysfunction. *The American Journal of Psychiatry* 153:503-512.

145. Hippocrates, as quoted in Burton R (1621): *The Anatomy of Melancholy*. The original appears in *The History of Epidemics, in Seven Books*. Trans. Samuel Farr.

146. Kitanaka J (2011): *Depression in Japan: Psychiatric Cures for a Society in Distress*. Princeton University Press.

147. Watters E (2010): *Crazy Like Us: The Globalization of the American Psyche*. Simon & Schuster.

148. Shorter E (1991): *From Paralysis to Fatigue: A History of Psychosomatic Illness in the Modern Era*. The Free Press.

149. Currin L (2005): Time trends in eating disorder incidence. *The British Journal of Psychiatry* 186(2):132-135.

150. Mostofsky E et al. (2012): Risk of Acute Myocardial Infarction After the Death of a Significant Person in One's Life. The determinants of myocardial infarction onset study. *Circulation* 125(3):491-6.

151. Plato, *Charmides*. Trans. Trevor J. Saunders.

152. Jung CG (1961): *Memories, Dreams, Reflections*, p140. Vantage Books.

153. Jung CG (1966): Two Essays on Analytical Psychology, par. 68. *Collected Works of C.G. Jung*, Volume 7. Princeton University Press.

154. Freud S (1895): *Studies in Hysteria*.

155. Freud S (1899): *The Interpretation of Dreams*.

156. Freud S (1927): *Die Zukunft einer Illusion (The Future of an Illusion)*. *Die Stimme des Intellekts ist leise, aber sie ruht nicht, ehe sie sich Gehör verschafft hat.*

157. Maslow AH (1943): A theory of human motivation. *Psychological Review* 50(4):370-96.

158. Aristotle: *Politics*, Bk. 8.

159. Sartre JP (1943): *Being and Nothingness: An Essay on Phenomenological Ontology*.

160. Tillich P (1952): *The Courage to Be*.

161. Shelley, PB (1818): *Ozymandias*.

6: Suicide and self-harm

162. Crane H (1932): *The Broken Tower*. This poem was written not long before Hart Crane committed suicide by jumping from the steamship SS Orizaba into the Gulf of Mexico.

163. Speech by the Deputy Prime Minister to the Mental Health Conference delivered on 19 January 2015. Transcript: https://www.gov.uk/government/speeches/nick-clegg-at-mental-health-conference

164. The British Psychological Society (2014): *Teen levels of self-harm on the increase*. News item published on 23/05/2014. http://www.bps.org.uk/news/teen-levels-self-harm-increase

165. Bacino L (2014): A World Health Organisation survey reveals that a fifth of 15-year-olds in England say they self-harmed over the past year. *The Guardian*, May 21,

2014. http://www.theguardian.com/society/2014/may/21/
shock-figures-self-harm-england-teenagers

166. Hawton K et al. (2002): Deliberate self harm in adolescents: self report survey in schools in England. *British Medical Journal* 325:1207.

167. Hawton K et al. (2012): *Self-Harm in Oxford 2012.* http://cebmh.warne.ox.ac.uk/csr/images/annualreport2012.pdf

168. Avevor, ED (2007): Self-harm—a culture bound syndrome? Ghana and UK experience. *The Psychiatrist* 31(9):357.

169. Speech by the Deputy Prime Minister delivered on 19 January 2015. Transcript: https://www.gov.uk/government/speeches/nick-clegg-at-mental-health-conference

170. Office for National Statistics: *Suicides in the United Kingdom, 2013 Registrations.* Published February 19, 2015. http://www.ons.gov.uk/ons/dcp171778_395145.pdf

171. World Health Organization (2012): Global Health Observatory data for suicide. http://www.who.int/gho/mental_health/en/

172. Goethe JW (1774): *The Sorrows of Young Werther.*

173. Salib E (2003): Effects of 11 September 2001 in suicide and homicide in England and Wales. *The British Journal of Psychiatry* 183:207-212.

174. Office for National Statistics: *Suicides in the United Kingdom, 2013 Registrations.* Published February 19, 2015. http://www.ons.gov.uk/ons/dcp171778_395145.pdf

175. Hume D (1783): *Essays on Suicide and the Immortality of the Soul.*

176. Sartre JP (1952): *Saint Genet, comédien et martyr (Saint Genet, Actor and Martyr),* Bk. 2.

177. Hume D (1783): *Essays on Suicide and the Immortality of the Soul.*

178. Pliny the Elder (c. 77): *Natural History*, Bk 2, Ch 7. *Deus non sibi potest mortem consciscere si velit, quod homini dedit optimum in tantis vitæ pœnis.*

179. Nagel T (1970): Death. *Noûs* 4(1):73-80.

Epilogue

180. Gide A (1894): *Journal 1889-1939*, Septembre 1894. Trans. Neel Burton. *Les choses les plus belles sont celles que souffle la folie et qu'écrit la raison. Il faut demeurer entre les deux, tout près de la folie quand on rêve, tout près de la raison quand on écrit.*

By the same author

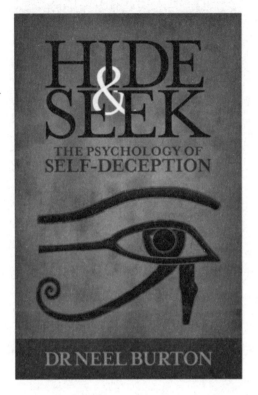

Hide and Seek, The Psychology of Self-Deception
ISBN 978-0-9560353-6-3

Self-deception is common and universal, and the cause of most human tragedies. Of course, the science of self-deception can help us to live better and get more out of life. But it can also cast a murky light on human nature and the human condition, for example, on such exclusively human phenomena as anger, depression, fear, pity, pride, dream making, love making, and god making, not to forget age-old philosophical problems such as selfhood, virtue, happiness, and the good life. Nothing could possibly be more important.

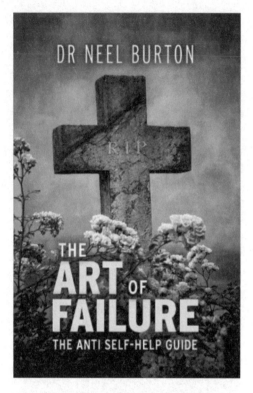

The Art of Failure, The Anti Self-Help Guide
ISBN 978-0-9560353-3-2

We spend most of our time and energy chasing success, such that we have little left over for thinking and feeling, being and relating. As a result, we fail in the deepest possible way. We fail as human beings.

The Art of Failure explores what it means to be successful, and how, if at all, true success can be achieved.

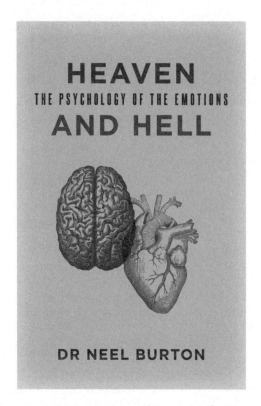

Heaven and Hell, The Psychology of the Emotions
ISBN 978-0-9929127-2-7

Today more than ever, the education doled out in classrooms is cold and cognitive. But, once outside, it is our uneducated emotions that move us, hold us back, and lead us astray. It is, at first and at last, our emotions that determine our choice of profession, partner, and politics, and our relation to money, sex, and religion. Nothing can make us feel more alive, or more human, than our emotions, or hurt us more.

Yet many people lumber through life without giving full consideration to their emotions, partly because our empirical, materialistic culture does not encourage it or even make it seem possible, and partly because it requires unusual strength to gaze into the abyss of our deepest drives, needs, and fears.

This book proposed to do just that, examining over 25 emotions ranging from lust to love and humility to humiliation, and drawing some useful and surprising conclusions along the way.

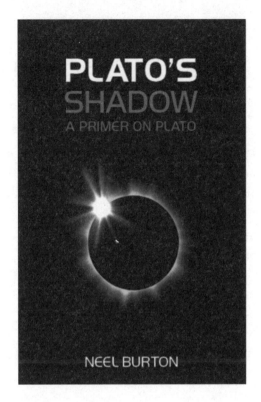

Plato's Shadow – A Primer on Plato
ISBN 978-0-9560353-2-5

Plato thought that only philosophy could bring true understanding, since it alone examines the presuppositions and assumptions that other subjects merely take for granted. He conceived of philosophy as a single discipline defined by a distinctive intellectual method, and capable of carrying human thought far beyond the realms of common sense or everyday experience. The unrivalled scope and incisiveness of his writings as well as their enduring aesthetic and emotional appeal have captured the hearts and minds of generation after generation of readers. Unlike the thinkers who came before him, Plato never spoke with his own voice. Instead, he presented readers with a variety of perspectives to engage with, leaving them free to reach their own, sometimes radically different, conclusions. 'No one,' he said, 'ever teaches well who wants to teach, or governs well who wants to govern.'

This book provides the student and general reader with a comprehensive overview of Plato's thought. It includes an introduction to the life and times of Plato and – for the first time – a précis of each of his dialogues, among which the Apology, Laches, Gorgias, Symposium, Phaedrus, Phaedo, Meno, Timaeus, Theaetetus, Republic, and 17 others.

Index